the ABCs of vitamins, minerals, and natural foods

JOHN PAUL LATOUR

AN
ARC
BOOK

ARCO PUBLISHING COMPANY, INC.

219 Park Avenue South, New York, N.Y. 10003

Third Printing, 1977

Published by Arco Publishing Company, Inc.
219 Park Avenue South, New York, N.Y. 10003

Library of Congress Catalog Card Number 72–3503
ISBN 0–668–02655–3

Printed in the United States of America

CONTENTS

Foreword

To stay young, never grow old and always remain healthy are legitimate wishes most of us cherish dearly. Although the desire for eternal life must still remain a dream, today we are fortunate that the gift of perfect health lies within reach of every one of us. In the past, primitive man had to spend most of his time and energy trying to acquire sufficient food just to stay alive. Individuals who always had nourishment were considered wealthy then, and obesity was regarded as a mark of distinction.

As time went on, advances in agriculture provided abundant food for those living in wealthier nations. No longer satisfied to merely overcome his hunger, man demanded foods which were nourishing, good tasting and attractive as well. Cooking developed into a fine art. Scientists began to study the effects of particular foods upon man, and today, as we accumulate more and more knowledge, dietetics has become a very exact science. Information about the nature of essential components in our

1

foods, about their specific effects upon our health, and about their importance in our diet, is knowledge available to everyone now.

However, modern advances in agriculture and food processing have introduced some problems as well. Because the preparation and distribution of our food represents a 13-billion-dollar-a-year industry, the requirements of efficiency and packaging sometimes may work against the principles of proper nutrition. The more modern man strays from nature, the more imbalances he creates in his body chemistry. Fortunately, though, by understanding the needs of our bodies we can at least, in part, control our destiny in a scientific manner. Chemistry has very stable laws which apply to our bodies as well, for foods can be considered chemicals acting on our bodies. Nutrition studies the effects of these foods on our bodies. We have the choice of selecting foods to benefit our health instead of foods detrimental to us. The choice is not difficult to make, once we understand the principles of body health.

The purpose of this book is to provide the basic knowledge about foods, vitamins, minerals and poisons in the clearest and most accessible form, and to elucidate some of the questions which still surround the field of health and nutrition. The findings reported here are based upon the most modern research into the biological and enzymatic processes of food metabolism; all information is accurate, up to date, and derived from official sources.

I have organized this book as a reference work about vitamins, minerals, and food so that specific information may be easily looked up when questions arise. The final chapter deals with poisons and poisonous plants and describes emergency measures one may take immediately, before treatment is completed by a physician or at a hospital.

Every consideration has been taken to make this book enjoyable and convenient to use as well as informative. It is my hope that your readings here will benefit you in your quest for a healthier way of life.

John Paul Latour   B. Phm. Université de Montreal
B. Ph. University of the Pacific

1

Vitamins

Vitamins are a group of chemicals which are essential for normal growth and the maintenance of health in man. For the most part, they cannot be manufactured by the body. First, they are synthesized by bacteria in the soil; then, plants absorb them from the soil, and man feeds on the plants containing vitamins. Vitamins are stored mainly in the glands, the liver and the kidneys.

The absence of any one vitamin in the diet causes specific symptoms and results in "deficiency diseases." The study of vitamins is done by observing animals which are fed a diet containing every vitamin except the one being studied. Whatever symptoms the vitamin-deficient animal shows, point to the effects of the vitamin under investigation.

The letters assigned to vitamins have nothing to do with their chemistry but are merely used for identification purposes. Vitamins are classified according to their solubility. Some vitamins are lipo-soluble (soluble in oil) such as vitamins, A D, E and K. Other vitamins are hydro-soluble (soluble in water); the B complex and C vitamins belong to this group. The solubility of vitamins is important in manufacturing and also in cooking, when, for instance, all of the water soluble vitamins may be lost if the water used to cook foods containing them is discarded. Vitamins can be destroyed by air, light, overcooking of foods or excessive heat.

There has been some exaggeration concerning the destruction of vitamins in the preparation of manufactured foods, but caution is still called for. Processes used in drying fruits and smoking fish reduce much of the vitamin content of these foods. Canning, now done with minimum exposure to air, is at least partially successful in avoiding oxidation, which destroys vitamins. Rapid and complete freezing is the one method which we know of that preserves all the vitamins in foods.

Ideally, we should eat foods soon after they are prepared. But even if we do, and follow all the precautions for preserving the vitamins in our food, it still may be difficult to maintain the proper nutritional balance. Fortunately, vitamin supplements, especially those containing minerals as well, are available and relatively inexpensive. When we consider the health advantages of a balanced diet, the minimal added cost to our budgets for these supplements seems well worthwhile. Minerals should not be underestimated in all the recent concern about nutrition, for they are responsible for countless enzymatic reactions and for the transmission of nerve impulses and muscle activity. Minerals will be discussed at length in Chapter 2.

Before proceeding to the discussion of individual vitamins we should first consider some pertinent information about dosage, different forms, and relative costs of vitamins.

Dosage

The average dose estimated to maintain health for each vitamin is established by the National Research Council and is a numerical figure which expresses either United States Pharmacopeia units (U.S.P. Units), International Units (I.U.), or parts of a gram, usually milligrams (one thousandth of a gram), abbreviated mg, or one thousandth of a milligram (or microgram, one millionth of a gram), abbreviated mcgm. This average dose is called the minimum daily requirement (M.D.R.). This M.D.R. has not been established for all vitamins and minerals, for some are known to be needed in health maintenance but their quantities have not been established scientifically. Even when a dosage can be established, it may vary slightly with any individual.

Occasionally, therapeutic formulas of vitamins are recommended. These constitute dosages far above the Minimum Daily Requirements and should not be taken over long periods of time. They often do not have the dramatic effect expected of them; in fact, they can even be damaging. For example, some therapeutic formulas call for 25,000 units of vitamin A. This alone may burden the liver and damage the eyesight. Granted that a few people are vitamin resistant and will not respond readily to vitamins, but even they should use caution and not overdose themselves over long periods. Their problem may be one of difficulty in absorption rather than resistance, unless there is a hormonal imbalance.

Natural or Synthetic Vitamins

Natural vitamins are not always natural even if the label says so. Some contain a fair amount of synthetics. In any event, your expectations from these natural products are probably unrealistic. For example, there is an unsubstantiated claim that natural vitamin C does more than ascorbic acid. The active part of vitamin C *is* ascorbic acid. There is also a problem of size. A 100 mg natural vitamin C tablet is easy to swallow, but a 250 or 500 mg tablet would look more like half a ping-pong ball, and who could swallow that? Therefore, the manufacturers have to add ascorbic acid to natural vitamin C. Furthermore, there are not enough rose hips or cherry hips, two natural sources of vitamin C, to supply the market.

On the other hand, some vitamins are cheaper to obtain from natural sources—*e.g.*, the vitamins of the B complex—so there is no need to synthesize them. Vitamin A from natural sources has frequently produced allergic reactions, so the synthetic vitamin A is to be preferred over the natural. It seems then, that there is no rule about natural or synthetic vitamins which could apply to all.

Dosage Forms

The purpose of pharmacy is to make drugs and medications available to a patient in a form that he can use. For babies we have concentrated solutions which can be administered from a dropper. For children, we have syrups less concentrated than baby drops, which can be given by the teaspoonful. Older children can take the chewable tablets until they are ready for the swallow-type tablets which adults take. There is no true advantage in taking either a pill or a powder or a liquid form of vitamins, for absorption will take place at one stage or another in the digestive process.

Fortunately, in this country the Food and Drug Administration keeps close control on the production of vitamin supplements to protect the public against fraud. There are standards set by the F.D.A. to control the quality and compounding of vitamins and the purity of dyes used in producing them. Usually, manufacturers set their own standards, which are higher than those of the F.D.A. This is especially true of the bigger manufacturers, who stand to lose their reputation should they take risks in their manufacturing operation.

When Should Vitamins Be Taken?

If you have a one-a-day type vitamin-mineral formula, it is best taken in the earlier part of the day with or after breakfast. Should your stomach tend to upset easily, try taking your daily supplement with your biggest meal. If you still get stomach upsets, try taking vitamins only, without minerals; this may be your solution. Between meals, you can take vitamin C and calcium, which are not present in sufficient amount in the normal diet to give a decent supply to anybody. Vitamin E also should be taken between meals. I mention vitamin C and E and calcium because these three elements are not supplied adequately even in therapeutic formulas.

How Long Should You Take Supplements?

Unless you grow your own food, raise your own cattle and poultry, bake your own bread and guarantee the vitamin content of your foods, then you should take supplements forever.

Cost of Vitamins

As a rule, you will save money by buying a large size, so you should figure out how many you will use in a year; but I would not buy more than a year's supply of any vitamin, for the opening and closing of the container tends to let in air, and oxidation or rancidity may occur. (The expiration date is also being printed on the label by major drug firms producing vitamin-mineral supplements.) On a per dose basis, it costs more to buy liquid drops or syrup than tablets of vitamins. The chewable vitamins are slightly more than the swallow-type tablets. The vitamin-mineral type is hardly more costly than the vitamin only type, and the advantages of getting these essential minerals is worth the slight extra cost.

Which Vitamins

Formulas vary with manufacturers mainly because they use different authorities or review their formulations constantly. I have compiled an average taken from the main manufacturers' formulas in the U.S. Here is the average daily dosage for infants up to six years of age:

Vitamin A: 5000 units
Vitamin D: 400 units
Vitamin B-1: 1 mg

Vitamin B-2: 1.2 mg
Vitamin B-6: 1 mg
Vitamin C: 60 mg
Vitamin B-12: 2 mcgms
Vitamin E: 10 I.U.
Pantothenic acid: 5 mg
Iron: 10 mg
Niacin: 10 mg

A few years ago the B complex and vitamin E were not considered essential, but times have changed and today's babies benefit greatly from accumulated experience in the field of nutrition. Iron, which is not needed in a newborn until he is four to six weeks old, is not found in milk and, therefore, should be supplemented after that age.

The formulas above and below are far above the M.D.R. set by the National Research Council for many reasons, but mainly because absorption often is impaired and the quantity ingested has to be far greater than the quantity you want to get in the circulation. Below is an adult formulation available commercially in major brands. The advised daily dosage is one tablet for children six to twelve years old, two tablets for age group twelve to fifteen, and three tablets daily for fifteen years old and up.

Vitamin A: 5000 units
Vitamin D: 400 units
Vitamin B-1: 2.5 mg
Vitamin B-2: 2.5 mg
Vitamin B-6: 0.5 mg
Vitamin B-12: 5 mcg
Vitamin C: 50 mg

ate: 5 mg

ng

Io. .g
Coppe. .g
Calcium: 35 mg
Magnesium: 6 mg
Potassium: 10 mg

The only supplementations which I find useful would be the following:

Calcium: 20 grains taken 3 times daily.
Vitamin E: 100 units taken 2 to 4 times daily.
Magnesium: 30 mg taken twice a day.
Pantothenic acid: 50 mg taken 3 times daily.

It is cheaper to buy the available formulation of vitamins and minerals above and supplement separately the calcium, vitamin E, magnesium and panthothenic acid, which are not adequate in any way. You may read about these 4 elements later under their separate headings.

VITAMIN A

Vitamin A is essential for the maintenance of healthy tissue structure, mainly the skin and the gums. It promotes normal growth and sound teeth and maintains acute vision. Extensive studies made during World War II revealed that it was of great value in helping pilots see in semi-darkness. It activates the photoreceptors on the retina of the eyes, making them more sensitive to light of low intensity. Vitamin A is also used to correct dry skin, because it allows oil-soluble proteins to remain in the cells of the skin. This same action takes place on the epithelial tissues of the eyes, nose, mouth, throat and throughout the entire breathing, digestive and genitourinary systems. The sensitive tissues of these organs are highly prone to bacterial invasion. The bacterias secrete an enzyme which infects unprotected epithelial cells but will not damage tissues which have retained enough oil to be insulated against these invading organisms. Vitamin A is therefore advisable when repeated sore throats or frequent burning sensations upon voiding urine are experienced.

Vitamin A is also involved in bone growth, including the formation of protective tooth enamel. Oxidation within the body destroys vitamin A, but this process can be slowed down by taking vitamin E, which acts as an antioxidant. When using vitamins A and E, it is advisable to increase your consumption of vegetable oils, for these oils act as a vehicle for the vitamins, which are soluble in oil.

Constant use of mineral oil as a laxative can be detrimental because it will prevent the absorption of vitamins A and E as well as K, depriving the body the benefits of these vitamins. The damage will be far greater than simple constipation.

Good food sources of vitamin A are mainly fish liver oils, egg yolks, dairy products, liver, kidney and green leafy vegetables. Such foods should be eaten soon after cooking, for exposure to the air will oxidize and inactivate the vitamin A they contain.

The National Research Council recommends a daily dose of vitamin A which varies from 1,500 units for children up to 8,000 units in pregnancy and lactation. Therapeutic doses of 25,000 to 100,000 units per day should not be taken for periods longer than two weeks and care should be exercised to watch for toxic symptoms. Toxicity is shown by irritability, loss of appetite, loss of hair and vision damage along with tenderness of the extremities of the toes and fingers. The skin will also become dry at times. Discontinuing the high use of vitamin A usually will rectify these symptoms before any permanent liver or kidney damage is done.

THE B COMPLEX VITAMINS

The B complex vitamins are usually found together in the same foods. These vitamins comprise two groups depending on their activity: those which release energy from foods and those involved in the formation of red blood cells (hematopoietics). The energy-releasing factors include thiamine, niacin, riboflavin, biotin and pantothenic acid. The hematopoietics (red blood builders) are folic acid and B-12. Pyridoxine could belong to either group.

The B vitamins which release energy from foods are all involved in the absorption process of nutrition which takes place throughout the gastro-intestinal tract. The oxidation of food is necessary before the cell can utilize the energy that is released. This is done with the help of certain enzymes, which form simpler chemicals, which can be more easily absorbed, from the original amino-acids, proteins, fats and sugars of the food consumed.

The cells of the body perform assorted functions besides maintaining and reproducing themselves. Gland cells must discharge their secretions, nerve cells transmit impulses from the brain to the farthest extremities, muscle cells do mechanical work, intestinal cells sort the food which can be used by the body, and kidney cells differentiate between useful products and waste for excretion. The energy-releasing vitamins of the B complex group will be discussed individually in the following pages under separate headings.

The hematopoietic factors of the B complex replace the loss of red blood cells and correct their faulty formation. Without this factor, anemia results and worsens the condition of the whole system. Inadequate protein in the diet impairs the efficiency of the blood-forming elements and other tissues as well. Different types of anemias result from the different stages of cell development at which deprivation takes place. A blood test may indicate the appropriate measures that will remedy the situation.

All cells require iron for their function and more than half of the body's iron is in the hemoglobin of the red corpuscles. Iron is reabsorbed when the hemoglobin is replaced, but some losses do occur during menstruations, in surgery, accidents and ulcers. If these losses are excessive, this condition leads to iron deficiency anemia or simple anemia. This condition is often encountered in adolescents and in women during pregnancy and lactation. The symptoms are pallor, short breath, headache and dizziness leading to loss of appetite, nervousness and irritability. The skin may be dry and wrinkly and crack at the corners of the mouth. Growth may be impaired; also irregular menses may result. Infections occur easily and should be cleared before iron therapy can be instituted. A good diet with red meats, liver and beef or eggs is advised. If supplementation is required, iron therapy is highly effective and rapid in showing results. Recurrent anemias may suggest bleeding lesions (ulcers) and should be looked into.

Pernicious or secondary anemia used to be fatal before the advent of vitamin B-12 and of the intrinsic factor found in liver meat. Severe anemia usually precedes secondary anemia and is characterized by pearly eyes, paleness of the face, weakness, sore tongue and tingling of the hands and feet. B-12 allied with the intrinsic factor usually corrects this situation. It is thought that the underlying cause of pernicious anemia is not the lack of B-12 but the lack of intrinsic factor formation. When pernicious anemia does not respond to the B-12 and intrinsic factor treatment, folic acid is often administered. Folic acid needs vitamin C for its formation. In treating the macrocytic anemia of pregnancy with folic acid we have observed the eradication of brown spots which often develop on the skin as a result of anemia.

VITAMIN B—1

Thiamine, as vitamin B-1 is also called, is the anti-beriberi factor; thiamine deficiency causes neurological lesions in man. Lack of B-1 leads to dysfunction of the nervous system manifested in muscle weakness, loss of sensation at the extremities of the legs and arms, and, in extreme cases, paralysis. Heartbeat abnormalities may appear quite suddenly and cause tachycardia (fast heartbeat). There may also be muscle cramps and a burning sensation at the soles of the feet accompanied by ankle swelling and fatigue. Nervousness results and causes loss of appetite and ensuing constipation. Neuritis caused from lack of B-1 can also result in neuralgia, shingles and lumbago.

The main function of vitamin B-1 is to change glucose into glycogen, a ready source of energy which is stored in the liver. The needs for B-1 vary in proportion to the calories consumed, especially those calories from carbohydrates and sugars. When no more glycogen can be stored in the liver, the excess glucose will result in fat accumulated in the body. Heavy physical work requires more of a supply of B-1; the need is also increased during pregnancy and lactation. B-1 is often used to detoxicate excessive alcohol consumption and minimize obesity and liver impairment. Although obesity may not be healthy, a certain amount of fat is desirable to insulate the body against temperature changes and to give a better support to vital organs such as the kidneys and the bladder.

Vitamin B-1 may not have the whole answer to beri-beri and allied neurological symptoms. All of the B complex seems to be needed for a complete and lasting cure. Happily, the whole B complex group is found together in the same foods.

Beri-beri is uncommon in America, but in far eastern countries it occurs more often, especially in the first months of life. It starts with loss of appetite, vomiting and painful colic. Swelling and lack of respiration precede a grunting resembling a drowning of the vocal cords.

Later, the heartbeat is irregular, and nervousness, twitching and coma appear. Death follows. Each phase lasts a few hours, and the whole condition a day or two.

A diagnosis of thiamine deficiency is determined by examining the dietary habits of the patient. Poor nutrition, alcoholism, bad cooking habits and food faddism can result in lack of thiamine.

Vitamin B-1 is widely distributed in nature and may be found in whole grain cereals, milk, pork, liver, eggs, nuts, fish, dried yeast and enriched bread. Commercial bread has to be enriched with B-1 because the milling process of white flour removes this vitamin. So called "wheat bread" is merely white bread colored with caramel. One hundred percent whole wheat bread is the complete bread worthy of food connoisseurs.

Because vitamin B-1 is water soluble, a minimum amount of water should be used in cooking; overheating also destroys this vitamin.

A more recent attribute of vitamin B-1 has been to repel fleas and mosquitoes when taken in doses of 25 to 50 mg daily by mouth. The vitamin seems to impart a scent to body secretions which, although unnoticeable by other humans, is repugnant to these pests.

The daily established dose of B-1 is from 0.2 mg for infants to 1.5 mg for most adults, but because of absorption impairments common to most of us, the oral dose must be increased to between 10 and 100 mg daily. This vitamin is relatively nontoxic; daily doses as high as 500 mg taken for a month have not shown any bad symptoms. A few cases of sensitivity have resulted after repeated injections. Absorption is impaired by diarrhea, and great losses of B-1 result from the taking of diuretics (B-1 being water soluble). The taking of antibiotics also interferes with the body's natural production of B-1.

VITAMIN B–2

Vitamin B-2 is also called riboflavin, or vitamin G. B-2 is involved in the transport of hydrogen and the utilization of oxygen by the cells. The absence of riboflavin in the diet causes reddening of the lips and fissures at the corners of the mouth which don't heal normally. The mucous membranes of the eyelids and nostrils become pink and brittle, even rough, while the cornea of the eye shows small veins. The tongue takes on a magenta color, due to the blood being held in the taste buds. Exessive lacrimation and itching or burning of the eyes is also experienced. Dandruff frequently appears. The skin of the face may develop tiny globules of fat just under the surface of the skin. Pellagra (rough skin) and bloodshot eyes also occur.

The usual dose of riboflavin which will bring about remission of the above symptoms is 5 mg taken orally three times daily. The response should be within two weeks.

Riboflavin is abundant in nature and is also synthesized by our intestinal bacteria. Foods rich in vitamin B-2 include eggs, lean meats, liver, cheese, milk, leafy green vegetables and dried yeast.

The M.D.R. varies from 0.4 mg to 2 mg depending on age and conditions of pregnancy and lactation, when the needs increase. The therapeutic dose is 5 to 15 mg daily taken orally. Losses in cooking water are small because B-2 is not too soluble in water. Riboflavin is fairly stable when exposed to air and heat, but not when exposed to light, and it spoils when in solution. The toxic dose is far above the therapeutic dose of 15 mg per day, which makes it a very safe product to use.

NIACIN

Niacin is also called vitamin B-3 and vitamin PP (Pellagra-preventative). It is essential in respiration, where it acts in the oxidation of carbohydrates. Niacin is deeply involved in maintaining a normally functioning nervous system. Symptoms of lack of niacin include mental confusion, loss of appetite, insomnia, abdominal pain and diarrhea. Pellagra, a disease which involves the skin, the gastrointestinal tract and the nervous system, is relieved by niacin.

Niacin improves vision, and it acts as a vasodilator in increasing the circulation in the arms, legs and the brain. The feeling of warmth and even flushness experienced after taking niacin is not dangerous and usually vanishes after a few minutes. If this is intolerable, try taking niacinamide instead of niacin; the action is the same, since niacin becomes niacinamide in the body. Mental awareness is increased and problems of senility are reduced through usage of niacin. It also increases peripheral blood circulation, which may relieve ringing in the ears.

Good sources of niacin in foods are wheat germ, brewer's yeast, most meats, green peas, eggs and milk. The established needs range from 5 to 20 mg per day and are usually supplied by an average diet; but doses as high as 1000 mg with each meal have been used to treat alcoholism and dizziness. Under normal conditions, more moderate doses of 50 to 100 mg taken orally three times a day have been shown effective. High dosages of niacin should be avoided in presence of glaucoma, liver problems and peptic ulcers. The needs for niacin increase in proportion to muscular work. Niacin is rather stable in heat, air and light.

PANTOTHENIC ACID

Also known as vitamin B-5, pantothenic acid is involved in the release of energy from carbohydrates. It is really an enzyme but because its function is closely related to that of other members of the B complex group it is called vitamin B-5. It helps to maintain the blood sugar at a high level and has been shown to increase the capacity of the liver to store glycogen. Upon this capacity of the liver rests the ability of the body to resist stress. Pantothenic acid may be put to good use in cases of hypoglycemia, where the level of blood sugar keeps falling. Lack of pantothenic acid results in loss of coordination with muscular weakness of the hands and feet leading to degeneration of the spinal cord. Antisterility has not been confirmed positively but the vitamin does maintain the balance of male and female sex hormones. Deficiency of the vitamin can lead to abdominal cramps, headache, nausea, respiratory distress and even tetanus. Resistance to infection is also diminished. As seen from the above, all the B complex deficiencies lead to the same symptoms and can best be corrected by adding all of the B complex vitamins to the diet.

The usefulness of pantothenic acid in treating Addison's disease is related to the need of the adrenal glands, which secrete ACTH (hormone) and require pantothenic acid to function.

Vitamin B-5 is also involved in the defense systems of our body. The antigen-antibody reaction in experimental animals was found to stop when pantothenic acid was deficient in their diets. The rate of multiplication of certain bacilli also increased in rats deficient in the vitamin.

Another important area of action is in increasing stress resistance in human beings. Young men using the vitamin did not get shocked when immersed in ice-cold water, but those deficient in vitamin B-5 would shiver uncontrollably. More recent experiments on volunteers involve pantothenic acid and pyridoxine. It was found that deficiency of both vitamins eliminated the volunteers' immunity to typhoid and tetanus and lowered their available gamma globulin. Their immunity was restored after the two vitamins were replenished and vaccines given. This shows positively the relationship of the two vitamins with the ability of the body to produce antibodies.

If you should buy pantothenic acid supplements, it might be good to purchase the calcium salt of pantothenic acid called calcium pantothenate. This will increase your supply of calcium, which is so scantily distributed in foods. In normal diets, pantothenic acid is amply supplied by intestinal bacteria. It can be found in milk, eggs, liver, beef, pork, chicken, potatoes, tomatoes, nuts, broccoli and molasses.

The daily dose has not been officially established but ranges from 10 to 150 mg daily. Pantothenic acid is sensitive to heat, acids and alkalis, but is stable in neutral solutions.

PABA

Para Amino Benzoic Acid has the reputation of being the anti gray-hair factor. It has prevented gray hair when it has been tested on rats and mice, but the extent to which it works for human beings is still a highly controversial matter. The evidence points that it does work for man, but the effect has also been produced by folic acid, pantothenic acid and biotin—all of which are members of the B complex family. Only large doses of PABA have produced a reversion of gray hair to its natural color.

In man, PABA reduces the mortality rate in several types of rickettsial infections such as Rocky Mountain Spotted Fever, typhus, and other such diseases. The local action of PABA in ointment form has shown good results in some skin infections such as lupus erythematosus and other dermatitis. PABA also relieves the fever and joint pains of rheumatic fever. The use of aspirin and other salicylates increases the content of PABA in the blood. With cortisone, PABA alleviates rheumathoid arthritis. Ointments containing PABA protect the skin against the harmful effects of the sun's rays.

PABA is mainly restricted to prescription usage; it is usually nontoxic, but autopsies of acute cases of rheumatic fever treated with large doses of PABA have shown fatty changes in the liver, heart and kidneys.

VITAMIN B—6

Well known as pyridoxine, vitamin B-6 is responsible for the metabolism of fats, carbohydrates and proteins. It is a coenzyme which allows the buildup and destruction of proteins essential in the growing process. It controls the level of magnesium in the blood and tissues, which makes it responsible for a dozen enzymatic reactions essential in metabolism.

Deficiency of this vitamin in adults is shown by hair loss, swelling and behavioral changes, and in infants, by convulsive seizures. The latter was found through EKG tests on children who were fed a canned milk formula which contained no pyridoxine because it was lost in the sterilization process used in the manufacture. The children responded within minutes after administration of pyridoxine.

A very important action of pyridoxine is in the control it exercises on cholesterol; without B-6, cholesterol level rises without control, and the oxidation products of cholesterol are carcinogenic. Ten mg daily have relieved nausea of pregnancy and of X–Ray therapy. Vitamin B-6 helps in the buildup of tissues from amino-acids and lecithin.

The daily dose varies from 0.2 mg for infants to 2.5 mg for pregnant women, but the therapeutic dose of up to 150 mg per day does not present any undesirable side effects, which makes it a safe product to use.

Good food sources are liver and lean meats, wheat germ, green vegetables, potatoes, eggs, milk, corn, dried yeast and nuts. Vitamin B-6 is stable in heat but destroyed by light.

VITAMIN B–12

Cyanocobalamin, as vitamin B-12 is also known, is essential in the good functioning of all cells, especially those of the bone marrow, the nervous system and the digestive system. Its main usage has been to control pernicious anemia. As little as 1 mcg of it daily by injection has produced complete remission. As with cancer and diabetes, you can't hope to cure pernicious anemia, but you can control it in most cases.

Taken orally, vitamin B-12 has to be many times above the recommended 1 mcg daily for infants and 6 mcg daily for women during pregnancy or lactation. This is because the vitamin is destroyed to a great extent in the digestive tract, and absorption of the vitamin is impaired in many ways. Vitamin B-12 has been used in hepatitis because of its action in protein synthesis. In conjunction with folic acid, B-12 assures full maturation of the red blood cells. The most dramatic action of B-12 is still in controlling pernicious anemia, where the reticulocyte (immature red corpuscle) formation is restored within a week and the red and white cell count is back to normal within 5 or 6 weeks.

The best food sources of B-12 are mainly in animal meats, salt water fish, oysters and milk.

FOLIC ACID

The main role of folic acid is in the synthesis of nucleoproteins essential in the reproduction of human cells. By itself, folic acid can bring only an incomplete remission in pernicious anemia and will not prevent the progressing neurological lesions of this disease, but when combined with B-12, the improvement is dramatic. Folic acid absorption is impaired during the last few months of pregnancy and also in later years; during these periods, brown spots appear on the skin. Folic acid in supplements has been used to prevent or correct the appearance of the brown spots, very effectively in most cases.

The four oil soluble vitamins—A, D, E and K—cannot perform their individual actions without the presence of folic acid in the system. The sum result of lack of effectiveness of these vitamins is called sprue, which shows all the symptoms common to lack of each of these vitamins in the system. The regular use of laxatives and antacids impairs the absorption of folic acid. The need for folic acid is increased in alcoholism. Folic acid is easily absorbed orally or by injection. The dangerous dose is so far above the effective one that it is a safe product to use. It is, however, restricted to prescriptions because it can mask warning signals of other diseases.

Good food sources for folic acid are liver, whole meat, milk, spinach, lettuce and yeast. Normal diets supply the .02 to .8 mg needed daily. Folic acid is readily destroyed by heat or by exposure to sunlight.

BIOTIN

Biotin is also called Vitamin H or anti-egg-white-injury factor. Avidin, a substance found in egg whites, causes severe allergies and is neutralized by biotin. The main function of biotin is to synthesize lipids in the liver; it is also involved in the growth mechanism.

Lack of biotin in the diet has caused loss of hair, eczema, irregular heartbeat, physical weakness and mental depression. Biotin can be depleted in the system when the diet is frequently made up of raw egg whites.

Good food sources of biotin are meat, egg yolks, milk,

liver, kidney and most fresh vegetables. Intestinal fermentation also produces biotin. Normal average diets supply the 200 mg needed daily. Biotin is not destroyed by heat but oxidation will inactivate it.

VITAMIN C

Ascorbic acid, which is the active part of vitamin C, is well known for its anti-scurvy activity. Scurvy was prevalent among the early navigators. This disease involves the collagens, which are the connective tissues of the gums and other organs, and the intercellular substance of the blood vessels. Vitamin C is essential in cell respiration. It maintains the blood sugar at a normal level and prevents capillary fragility (breaking of small vessels). Vitamin C in doses of up to 3000 mg daily has been used to minimize the side effects of the common cold, and to quite a degree it does just that. However, the F.D.A., which regards ascorbic acid as a safe substance, warns that too much vitamin C can cause diarrhea. This may be dangerous, especially for elderly people and young children. It could even cause miscarriage in pregnancy. Scurvy of the newborn has also been observed when the mothers were on high doses of vitamin C. The offspring had to be supplemented soon after birth, for the mother was not supplying the high doses of the vitamin anymore. The acidifying effect of vitamin C on the urine of diabetics can also interfere in their treatment.

Vitamin C is used in conjunction with vitamin A in treating frequent colds. Their combined action is mainly on the collagens and the cellular tissue, which have an increased permeability; this prevents the antigens from invading the breathing system. The increased permeability of the cells resulting from the action of vitamin C is effective in preventing pyorrhea and other gum problems. Because of its direct action on the sex glands and the cortex, vitamin C has lowered edema (water retention) and corrected irregular metabolism. Healing is improved when the vitamin is well supplied, and arthritis to some degree is relieved quite rapidly.

The body cannot store vitamin C to any great degree, therefore frequent smaller doses are to be preferred over large massive doses.

Vitamin C is also an inhibitor of the ultra-violet light of the sun which produces changes in the proteins of the lens of the eye and of the skin. The sun accelerates the aging process of the tissues and vitamin C slows down this action. The ultra-violet light is responsible for tanning the skin and the amino acids oxidized in this fashion travel throughout the system effecting further oxidation. Consequently, the use of vitamin C in preventing needless oxidation of body proteins is a recommended practice. The combination of vitamin E as antioxidant and vitamin C as a reducer (oxygen acceptor) will show a synergistic action of antioxidation.

When taking iron it is a good idea to also take vitamin C; this keeps iron in its ferrous state, which is its most active form.

Vitamin C has several unexplored properties, much the same as other vitamins and minerals. There is no limit to its range of action, the latest of which involves schizophrenics who retain vitamin C in their system when compared to normal persons who eliminate vitamin C in a regular fashion in their urine.

Diets lacking in fresh fruits and vegetables usually lead to ascorbic acid deficiency, and we might bear in mind that improper storage or canning of fruits and vegetables harms their vitamin C content. Cooking also should be kept at a minimum. Destruction of vitamin C is accelerated by exposure to air and by the use of iron or copper pots in cooking. In solution, vitamin C is inactivated quickly; it is good to drink orange juice soon after preparation. High temperatures also destroy vitamin C. A minimum quantity of cooking water should be used in connection with this vitamin, since it is water soluble.

The main food sources of vitamin C are citrus fruits and their freshly prepared juices, tomatoes, peppers, cherries, cantalopes and most berries. The use of natural vitamin C from rose hips or cherry hips and other citrus vitamin products has not been proved to be superior to synthetic vitamin C. Any claim to the contrary is fraudulent.

The basic established daily dose for vitamin C varies from 35 to 60 mg; in cases of colds, 250 mg three times a day is common, but a dose as high as 3000 mg daily has been taken without toxicity. Caution should be used during pregnancy and with infants.

VITAMIN D

Vitamin D has been called the "Sunshine Vitamin," for it is ever present in the sun's rays. The biochemical mechanism of its action is still not fully known. It is an oil soluble vitamin; for it to be absorbed, some oil has to be present on the skin. Therefore, babies should not be bathed prior to exposure to the sun. One reason the American Indians had such beautiful white teeth is that bathing was not always readily available, so their natural secretions increased their absorption of the sun's rays.

This vitamin promotes the retention of calcium and phosphorus and maintains the concentration of these elements in the blood, thus allowing deposits of lime salts in the formation of bones. In toxic amounts, vitamin D depletes calcium and phosphorus from the bones. Overexposure to the sun can cause nausea and irritate the bronchi, the kidneys and the heart. Weight loss may follow. Vitamin C is also depleted and should be supplemented.

Lack of vitamin D during pregnancy leads to skeletal deformities in the offspring. Tooth development and bone growth are also impaired. In babies, there is a lack of calcium absorption, which leads to swollen wrists and ankles and to bad spine curvature. Irritability, restlessness and even tetanus develop, for calcium is essential in nerve and muscle function. In adults, irritability and constipation may set in. The regular use of mineral oil as a laxative impairs absorption of calcium and worsens the very condition for which it is taken.

The dose for vitamin D is 400 units a day for all ages and conditions. Food sources are scanty in nature but vitamin D may be obtained from eggs, fish, irradiated milk as well as from exposure to the sun. Overdosage should be avoided, especially in cases of nephritis and atherosclerosis or during pregnancy.

VITAMIN E

Vitamin E has become one of the most popular vitamins in recent years and for many good reasons. The first and most important reason lies in the fact that vitamin E is the answer to this ever-more hectic world man has created for himself. We are burning ourselves past the turning point. Our bodies are exposed to artificial means of living and, hence, oxidized at a rate far greater than our ancestors' were. The results affect our cells, which die prematurely or fail to mature fully. Vitamin E is an antioxidant which enables our tissues to perform efficiently on less oxygen. It makes full use of our capillary vessels by increasing their blood supply. This reserve of energy stored in the vessels is therefore made available for use in bodily functions. Recent experiments show that the life span of mice was increased by 40 percent when put on a diet of vitamin E concentrated foods.

How all this comes about is not fully known. Vitamin E may prevent free-radical damage, by increasing liver enzymes, by limiting food intake, or even by stimulating production of adrenal hormones; however it does its work, vitamin E has been justly popularized. Natural vitamin E has been reported somewhat more active than the synthetic, and this has been substantiated.

The action of vitamin E on cholesterol accumulated along the veins and arteries is such that the cholesterol is broken into smaller globules, tiny enough to feed the cells or be eliminated from the system. This is how heart patients benefit from vitamin E. It helps the circulatory system rid itself of the clogging effect of cholesterol, and restores a clean supply of blood to all the tissues. Numerous people have been taking 200 to 400 units a day after they had suffered two and three heart attacks. The results were amazing; after three or four weeks, not only did they feel better, but they could exercise, work and return to a normal way of life. Their chest pains were a thing of the past and their mental attitude was altogether different.

In a study by Dr. DiLuzio of Tulane School of Medicine, tests showed that a high cholesterol level is shown by a high level of "dienes" in the blood. Dienes are the resulting product of highly oxidized fats in the body. Such fats are formed even if the diet is high in polyunsaturates; they are toxic, just as animal fats are, because they form cholesterol. When vitamin E was added to the diet of volunteers with high dienes in their blood, Dr. DiLuzio found that the dienes were lowered, and when vitamin E was stopped, the dienes in the blood increased again. This is pretty conclusive, and at long last we have a chemical way to calibrate the action of vitamin E in the system. With so much potential, research is being increased in the field of vitamin E. Because it is such a natural product, vitamin E creates no imbalances within the body.

In another study, Dr. Horwitt of the University of Illinois showed that on a diet low in vitamin E the red blood cells ruptured easily. When vitamin E was restored, the capacity of the red cells to carry oxygen was increased; this shows that the antioxidant action of vitamin E lessens the need for the lungs to supply as much oxygen under the same conditions. Some experiments on lung cancer being conducted at present involve usage of vitamin E; the results are still inconclusive, but promising.

I have no doubt about vitamin E retarding the aging process by delaying the destruction of the cell's lipo-proteins (oil soluble proteins). On this subject, Dr. Tap-pel of the University of California said that the destruc-tion of fat by oxygen is "the basic deteriorative reaction" which can be slowed down by antioxidants such as vita-min E. Recently, Dr. Tappel showed evidence that vita-min E can protect the lungs against air pollution. It is my opinion that cancer can't be cured per se, but can be held back and even regressed by treating the symptoms, much the same as diabetes is controlled, but not cured, by insulin treatment.

In 1969 the American Academy of Pediatrics recom-mended that vitamin E be included in all infant formulas. This decision came after some premature infants who had been fed a special formula rich in cottonseed oil de-veloped irritability, skin lesions and changes in the red blood cells. When vitamin E was added to the diet, all the symptoms cleared up. Several more reports followed and confirmed these findings; vitamin E was then in-cluded in infant formulas.

Vitamin E in combination with methionine has been used to treat liver necrosis (the death of liver tissues); the antioxidant action of vitamin E allied with the lipo-tropic (fat carrier) effect of methionine gives both in-gredients the extra activity needed to act on the liver cells.

Vitamin E can be used as ointment or lotion (squeezed out of the capsule) on all types of eczemas, burns and post surgical scars, which heal with hardly a trace; proud flesh diminishes in size and is often repigmented, wounds heal better and quicker, cold sores vanish and psoriasis improves dramatically, especially if the vitamin is taken orally as well. This same beneficial action also occurs in the digestive tract; ulcers have been healed and intestinal irritability reduced.

The same effect is true of the urinary tract. When there is a burning sensation upon voiding urine and this condition seems to recur, a combination of 50,000 units daily of vitamin A and 400 units of vitamin E for a period of ten days gives excellent and lasting results in 75 percent of the cases. The same treatment also applies to frequent colds. Varicose veins also respond to this treatment, however, in this case vitamin A should not exceed 25,000 units daily; the two vitamins, A and E, prevent destruction of fats by allowing lipo-proteins to feed the tissues surrounding the varicosities, thus diminishing their water content. In many cases, the tissues have healed to the point of being unnoticeable.

Vitamin E has often been referred to as the "sex vitamin." Although there is no action on the libido, vitamin E does increase the motility of the sperm towards the ovum.

As we have mentioned, vitamin E has an effect on the capillary vessels, which benefit from a better blood supply and thus increase the body's stamina and raises the memory level.

Vitamin E is present in wheat germ oil and other unsaturated vegetable oils, in nuts, wheat germ, whole grain cereals and leafy green vegetables. The daily basic needs in human nutrition as established by the National Research Council vary from 3 units for infants up to 30 units for adults. These are international units, since there are no U.S.P. units. These doses are basic, but for therapeutic purposes the dosage may be as high as 1,600 units daily. This dose should not be taken over long periods, for although vitamin E has always been regarded as safe, some researchers have indicated that very large doses may cause decalcification of the bones by depleting phosphorus needed for bone growth and repair.

The usual dose for vitamin E in most cases varies between 200 and 400 units. This covers cases of hypercholesterolemia (high cholesterol), allergies, atherosclerosis, premature aging, recurring digestive and breathing difficulties, debility, lack of stamina, varicosities and circulation problems including ulcerated varicose veins, most of which have been discussed in the above paragraphs.

Vitamin E is stable in heat but easily oxidized in the air. In the presence of sunlight it is destroyed. Soft gelatin capsules are to be preferred to coated tablets, for gelatin will seal off the air and protect the contents of vitamin E with a wider margin of safety. Vitamin E is the most promising product, man has come across in recent years.

VITAMIN K

Vitamin K is needed for the formation in the liver of prothrombin, which, with calcium, thrombin and other factors, coagulates the blood. The absence of vitamin K will result in hemorrhages, internal as well as external. This has been shown in experiments on young chicks placed on a vitamin K deficient diet; they developed fatal bleeding from prolonged coagulation time. These hemorrhages can be spontaneous or chronic.

Newborns have a very low supply of vitamin K, which has to be supplemented if surgery is performed on them. Shortly after birth the baby is able to synthesize adequate amounts of vitamin K, and with a normal diet this will continue through his entire life.

The body's production of vitamin K takes place in the intestinal flora; therefore, the constant use of mineral oil as a laxative will deprive the system of its vitamin K supply as well as that of other oil soluble vitamins such as vitamins A, D and E. Other causes for depletion of vitamin K are diarrhea, sprue and ulcerative colitis. The prolonged use of antibiotics, as in acne treatments, also interferes with the intestinal production of vitamin K.

In foods, vitamin K is found mainly in green plants and hog liver, but intestinal bacterias are the main suppliers under normal diets. Yogurt favors this process. The daily needs are around 2 mg.

VITAMIN F

In this category we find the all-important essential fatty acids: linoleic, linolenic and arachidonic acids. These are the prerequisites for the formation in the body of prostaglandins, which are responsible for the maintenance and repair of the tissues forming the different organs of our body. Prostaglandins are active in small quantities, much the same as hormones and the other vitamins. They are manufactured by the body cells and every cell produces its own special prostaglandin. This production cannot take place without adequate amounts of essential fatty acids in the diet.

Linoleic and linolenic acids abound in nature and can be found in vegetable oils, whole grain cereals, seeds such as sunflower, pumpkin and watermelon seeds, and nuts, while arachidonic acid is converted in the body from linoleic acid. Prostaglandins are not available commercially but research has identified about twenty of them and is showing promising prospects for their usage.

Experiments on animals have shown that fat-free diets lead to skin lesions, infertility and impaired growth. A diet which includes essential fatty acids often avoids and corrects allergies, asthma, gastric ulcers and promotes healing. Because the lack of essential fatty acids is a diet deficiency, it is often hard to pinpoint the cause of these diseases, but adequate intake of these essential fatty acids leads to production of prostaglandins. Vitamin E and pyridoxine (vitamin B-6) also favor the production of prostaglandins.

Every cell in your body has need to maintain and repair itself, and by making certain that your diet includes these foods which allow formation of prostaglandins, you are allowing your tissues to repair themselves. It has been advanced that the usage of aspirin and other pain relievers interferes with prostaglandin production or even destroys prostaglandins. To this day we do not know how aspirin works, but one sure thing is that it does not cure the cause of arthritis and other degenerative diseases; because of its action on the cell itself, aspirin might even aggravate the disease. Because nature has ample supply of essential fatty acids, why not make certain that your

diet includes these foods which allow tissue repair and
maintenance—namely, unsaturated vegetable oils, whole
grain cereals and sunflower, pumpkin and other seeds.

For the benefit of those readers interested in complete-
ness, I am listing most vitamins known to date. All of
them have been thoroughly investigated and most have
some value in nutrition. Their nomenclature is followed
by a summary of their actions.

VITAMIN A GROUP

Vitamin A-1: Also called retinol or axerophtol.

Vitamin A-2: Also called dehydroretinol or dehydro-3-
retinol.

Vitamin A Acid: Known as retinoic acid.

Retinine-1: Also called retinol.

Retinine-2: Also called dehydroretinol and dehydro-3-
retinol.

VITAMIN B GROUP

Vitamin B: First known as water soluble B. Originally
thought to relieve beri-beri but was found to contain
many factors.

Vitamin B-Complex: Known as the B vitamins. Group
isolated from yeast, liver and other sources having B-
soluble vitamins.

Vitamin B-1: Called thiamine, aneurine, antineuritic factor, vitamin F. An anti-beri-beri factor.

Vitamin B-2: Also called riboflavin, vitamin G, lacto-
flavin, ovoflavin, hepatoflavin. Essential for cellular oxy-
dation and reduction.

Vitamin B-3: Known as filtrate factor and chick pellagra factor. Essential for the growth of pigeons; may be identical to pantothenic acid.

Vitamin B-4: Prevents muscular weakness in rats and chicks. May be a mixture of riboflavin and pyridoxine or of arginine and glycine.

Vitamin B-5: Needed for growth of pigeons; many possibly be niacin.

Vitamin B-6: Called pyridoxine, pyridoxal, pyridoxamine, pyridoxol, the eluate factor, the rat acrodynia factor, adermin, vitamin Y.

Vitamin B-7: Also called vitamin I, rice factor. A factor in rice polishings that avoids digestive disturbances in pigeons.

Vitaman B-8: Is adenylic acid. May not be a true vitamin, but helps in phosphate transfer.

Vitamin B-9: This number is not used because nine of the B vitamins were known when B-10 and B-11 became known.

Vitamin B-10: The chick feathering factor; probably folic acid and B-12.

Vitamin B-11: The chick growth factor; also probably a mixture of folic and B-12.

Vitamin B-12: Also called cobalamin and cyanocobalamin.

Vitamin B-12b: Is hydroxycobalamin.

Vitamin B-12c: Is nitritocobalamin.

All B-12's are the antipernicious anemia principle identical with the extrinsic factors, the erythrocite maturation factor and maybe the animal protein factor.

Vitamin B-13: May be lipoic acid, probably identical to

protogen. It is uncharacterized and was found in distiller's dried soluble. Promotes growth in rats.

Vitamin B-14: May be related to xanthopterin, an analog of folic acid.

Vitamin B-15: Known as pangamic acid. Eases oxygen uptake in anoxia in rabbits.

Vitamin B-c: Chick factor, identical with folic acid.

Vitamin B-p: Antiperosis factor for chicks. Replaceable by choline and manganese.

Vitamin B-t: Known as carnitine. Growth factor for insects.

Vitamin B-w: Another name for biotin.

Vitamin B-x: Name used for pantothenic acid and p-aminobenzoic acid.

Nicotinamide: Niacinamide, P–P factor, anti black-tongue factor. Prevents pellagra (rough skin).

Nicotinic acid: Also called niacin. Is converted to niacinamide in the body.

Pantothenic acid: Known as pantothen, filtrate factor, chick antidermatitis factor, factor II, antichromotrichia (anti-gray hair) factor. Prevents dermatitis in chicks and achromotrichia in rats.

Biotin: Also called anti-egg white injury factor, vitamin H, coenzyme R, bios II, factor S, factor W, factor X. Cures alopecia and "spectacle eye" in rats fed a diet free of biotin but heavy in egg whites.

Choline: Also called bilineurine. Needed for transmethylation and also is a lipotropic agent.

Inositol: Known also as inosite, bios I, mouse antialopecia factor, muscle sugar. Prevents alopecia and "spectacle eye" in some animals. Lipotropic agent.

P-aminobenzoic acid: Abbreviated PAPA. Prevents gray
hair in rats and promotes growth in chicks.

Folic acid: Also called pteroyl glutamic acid (PGA),
folacin, vitamin M, vitamin Bc, factor U, lactobacillus
casei factor, norite eluate factor, factor M, vitamin
B-10, vitamin B-11. Is needed for growth and blood
formation.

Folinic acid: The citrovorum factor. A biologically active
form of folic acid.

VITAMIN C GROUP

Vitamin C: Ascorbic acid, cevitamic acid. Antiscorbutic
factor.

Vitamin C-2: Same as with vitamin J.

VITAMIN D GROUP

Vitamin D: Antirachitic factor.

Vitamin D-2: Known as calciferol, viosterol, irradiated
ergosterol, ergocalciferol.

Vitamin D-3: Known as cholecalciferol and irradiated
7-dehydrocholesterol.

VITAMIN E GROUP

Vitamin E: May be alpha or mixed tocopherols. Antisterility factor, antioxidant.

OTHER VITAMINS

Vitamin F: Obsolete name for essential fatty acids. Also
the old name for thiamine.

Vitamin G: Obsolete name for riboflavin.

Vitamin H: Obsolete name for biotin.

Vitamin I: Vitamin B-7.

Vitamin J: Also called vitamin C-2. Supposed to be an antipneumonia principle.

Vitamin K: Danish name for coagulation vitamin. Blood clotting factor. Anti-hemorrhagic factor.

Vitamin K-1: Also called phylloquinone.

Vitamin K-2: Also known as farnoquinone.

Vitamin L-1: Necessary for lactation. Related to anthranilic acid.

Vitamin L-2: Also needed for lactation. Related to adenosine.

Vitamin M: Obsolete name of folic acid.

Vitamin N: Factors from brain and stomach, supposedly cancer inhibitors. Now obsolete.

Vitamin P: Group of factors that decrease capillary fragility. Also known as citrin, bioflavonoids, citrus vitamin products, permeability factors. Not really considered as vitamins.

Rutin: One of the vitamin P factors.

Vitamin R: Promotes bacterial growth. Possibly in the folic acid group.

Vitamin S: Promotes bacterial growth, probably biotin. Applied to chick growth factor.

Vitamin T: Reported to improve protein assimilation in rats and produce giant insects. Also known as termite factor.

Vitamin U: Promotes bacterial growth. Probably one of the folic acid group. Also applied to a factor in cabbage juice that may correct peptic ulcers.

Vitamin V: Promotes bacterial growth. Possibly dipho-
sphopyridine nucleotide, the nicotinamide enzyme.

Vitamin W: Probably biotin. Promotes bacterial growth.

Vitamin X: Probably biotin. Promotes bacterial growth.

Vitamin Y: Possibly identical with pyridoxine.

2

Minerals and Water

WATER

About 65 per cent of the body weight is water. Most chemical reactions necessary to maintain life take place in water. It is estimated that 13 per cent of this water is lost each day through urination, perspiration and the feces. At this rate, dehydration would occur within four to five days. Therefore it takes around 2½ quarts of water to replenish the losses. This water comes from drinking water, tea, milk, juices and from the oxygenation of hydrogenated compounds. Thirst is the usual sign of the need for water, but if the urine has a strong odor or is of a deeper color than usual, this is also a sign of need for water. The kidneys function better when ample water is supplied. Conversely, frequent urination, especially if there is a burning sensation, and constant thirst are also warning signals, possibly of diabetes. When water is lost in hot weather, one should also replenish the lost salt dissolved in perspiration. Water intoxication results sometimes when only the water is replaced, and not the salt.

The kidney function is regulated by hormones. This is why there are great variations of weight before and after menstruation. Because birth control pills influence the hormones, they also exert a control on water-retention hormones. Effective diuretics are not available without prescriptions, and for good reasons. Diuretics stimulate the kidneys to lose extra water, but they also eliminate large amounts of potassium dissolved in this excreted water. This leads to muscle weakness and in the long run to losses of water-soluble vitamins; hence there is a general feeling of sluggishness which worsens with time.

The use of salt substitutes containing potassium is a good way to replace potassium losses caused by diuretics. Supplementation of the B complex and C vitamins, which are water soluble, may be of value to the person taking diuretics. Water retention is best avoided by restricting salty foods, spices and other salts in the diet (salts of sodium).

MINERALS

The role of minerals in nutrition has been established but seems to be undervalued when compared to vitamins. Too little has been said about minerals and it is so easy to deplete the diet of minerals, for instance, merely by discarding the cooking water of your vegetables. Using little water or a pressure cooker may prevent the losses of minerals in food. Much remains to be learned about minerals: What enzymatic reactions do they trigger, at what level do they act in the system, what systems do they affect and to what extent?

Minimum daily requirements have been established for Calcium, Iodine, Iron, Magnesium, and Phosphorous, but several more minerals are known to be essential for the normal functioning of the system, such as Manganese, Potassium, Sodium, Copper and Zinc. For these, however, no minimum has been established, so only an approximate dosage can be given. It is a matter more of ignorance than finance when well-to-do and seemingly clever people with sufficient income buy or prepare foods without essential minerals. When buying vitamin supplements, why not get the formulas with minerals added: they cost hardly any more than the vitamins alone. This supplementation of vitamins with the minerals is more imperative than ever, and here is the reason: Cultivation of fruits and vegetables is becoming more commercialized. The use of chemical fertilizers gives us faster and bigger crops, but this is at the expense of the soil which is depleted of its humus, and humus is responsible for keeping minerals in solution in the soil for the plants to absorb. If the minerals are not in solution, the plants will grow, but without any minerals, thus depriving us of our main source of these essential nutrients. Therefore, we need to supplement minerals in our vitamin formulas.

CALCIUM

Never has such an inexpensive yet important element been so undervalued. Calcium is necessary in bone growth and tooth maturation. It is involved in the blood clotting mechanism and is essential to nerve transmission and muscle contraction. A lack of calcium in the system causes irritability, particularly noticeable in growing children, for their need is especially high at that stage of development.

Children of growing age have a sweet tooth, which impairs calcium absorption, for sweets require large amounts of gastric juices in their digestion, and so does calcium. This is the real reason why sweets are bad for your teeth, because calcium absorption is impaired. Calcium can relieve premenstrual tension and cramps by aiding muscle contraction in much the same way it alleviates leg cramps. The relief of night leg cramps can be attained by taking 5 or 10 grains of quinine, but the cure rests mainly in an adequate supply of calcium in the diet. Calcium lactate has been used successfully as an anticonvulsant. The relief of colitis and spastic constipation is also effected by adequate calcium intake. One common occurence which can happen at any age is sudden dental decay accompanied by insomnia and skin disorders; all are due to a lack of calcium.

The daily need for calcium is established at 0.4 to 1.4 gm daily, but many times those quantities have to be ingested, for calcium is not the most soluble element and has to be available constantly for absorption in the digestive tract. The needs obviously are greater during pregnancy and lactation and during the growing years of twelve to sixteen years.

Normal diets do not oversupply calcium. Milk is a good source and one full quart a day seems adequate. Irradiated milk has vitamin D added, which helps calcium absorption. Some calcium preparations have vitamin D or viosterol added to help calcium absorption. Yogurt is an excellent source of calcium. Supplements of calcium are inexpensive and worth every penny. A good value when buying calcium supplements is to get calcium phosphate, because this product supplies both calcium and phosphorous. The metabolism of calcium is dependant upon vitamins A, B complex, C and D, and its assimilation rests on phosphorous and iron. Calcium is indeed inexpensive to supply in tablet form and still remains scanty in foods. It is best absorbed if taken between meals and a dosage of 20 grains two or three times daily is the optimum way to ingest calcium.

FLUORINE

Fluorine and its salts, the fluorides, are useful in bone growth and hardening. Fluorine benefits the teeth by increasing the resistance of the enamel to acids and hence to cavities. The drinking water in some areas is supplemented with fluorine; if it is not, then you must decide if there is a need to supplement fluorine as well as vitamins for your children. If the content is ½ PPM (part per million) of fluorine in your water supply, then the supplement should be around 0.5 mg daily, usually given in a chewable form because of the beneficial local action of fluorine on the teeth themselves. This supplement should be given especially during the ages of one to fourteen, when the crowns of the teeth are being formed.

Overdosage of fluorine should be avoided, for it will cause a brown mottling on the teeth, making them unsightly. This has happened frequently in northern Texas and New Mexico, where fluorine is present up to 3 PPM in the natural sources of drinking water.

The most effective way to prevent frequent recurring

tooth decay is to use old fashioned dental floss, preferably unwaxed. The theory is that most decay occurs between the teeth where tooth brushes can't always reach easily, and this is where bacteria multiply rapidly. When you disturb these bacterial beds with dental floss, their reproduction is prevented and decay avoided.

Fluorine has also been used in trying to delay arteriosclerosis, but this is still under investigation. At present, fluorine in large doses is being used under close medical supervision to treat osteoporesis (hollow bone formation).

Great controversy exists on the subject of fluoridation, and nutritionists argue that although the Food and Drug Administration endorses fluorinating our drinking water supplies, fluorine is still a poison. (In highly concentrated amounts, fluorine is indeed a violent poison.) Also, some fluorinating programs are conducted in a haphazard way, and furthermore, no two persons drink the same amount of water. Nutritionists have a good case and maybe they will be proven right, for the cure might well be worse than the ill; deeper penetration of fluorine in the body's system may interfere with tissue differentiation and bone growth. This is still being investigated and until there is further evidence I will withhold my opinion on the subject. In my house, we have mineralized bottled water and the fluorine supplied is given in a chewable vitamin-with-fluoride tablet containing 0.5 mg of fluoride.

IODINE

Iodine is essential for the proper functioning of the thyroid gland. Thyroid secretions affect the growth of the individual, both physically and mentally. Reproductive glands also are affected by thyroid. Should there be a lack of iodine in the diet, the thyroid gland will work harder, trying to secrete adequate amounts of thyroid hormone, and it will enlarge. This condition is known as goitre. Sometimes goitre can be alleviated by supplementing iodine, but surgery is the usual route.

Drinking water supplies some iodine, as do vegetables grown in soils containing iodine. The best source is iodized table salt and most sea foods. The daily needs are around 0.1 mg.

The color of the hair and its texture are also greatly affected by iodine. Some anemias have been traced to a lack of iodine in the diet. During pregnancy there is a crucial need for this mineral, for without iodine the fetus may be affected physically and mentally. Iodine is lost in the urine and perspiration and therefore should be replenished daily. For most people iodized salt is the best source, but again, when buying vitamins, get the vitamins with minerals combination. You can't afford to be without minerals.

IRON

Iron is a component of the hemoglobin which, with the help of some enzymes, carries oxygen to the cells. Although our blood is completely replaced about three times each year, the iron is reabsorbed and used again in newly formed hemoglobin. The yellow and green pigments of the bile are formed from hemoglobin.

Losses of iron are minor in the feces. Most iron losses

are from bleeding ulcers, heavy menses, cancer of the colon and the stomach, or bleeding from the urinary tract. The absence of iron in the diet, especially when losses are heavy, will cause simple anemia, which is easily corrected by supplementing the diet with iron preparations.

Newborn babies need no iron for the first two or three months, but after that time they should be given foods containing iron, such as egg yolks, fruits and green vegetables. Milk cannot supply iron in adequate amounts. Older children can get iron from meats, molasses, green vegetables, fruits, nuts and whole grain cereals.

The need for iron as established by the National Research Council varies daily from 6 to 18 mg, but because iron is absorbed poorly, the supplement must be far above that; somewhere around 300 mg three times daily is a universally accepted dosage. Iron may cause stomach upsets and intestinal disturbances, (diarrhea or constipation); these side effects can be avoided by taking the slow release or long acting forms of iron. Taking iron with meals slows down its absorption and diminishes its side effects. The combination of vitamin C with iron keeps the iron in its most active (ferrous) form.

Symptoms of lack of iron include paleness of the face, shortness of breath, brittle nails and palpitations of the heart. Mentally, one may experience forgetfulness and depression. Over the years I have seen girls in their teens who would get sessions of pimples in the face, especially at the time of their menses. I suggested iron and in most cases it did the trick after only one or two months after they started taking iron. Copper and other minerals are needed for iron to perform fully in its blood-building function. When buying vitamins, get the mineral-vitamin combination; the few pennies per 100 tablets are well spent.

MAGNESIUM

Magnesium is essential in the transmission of brain impulses through the nerves and in muscle contraction. The lack of magnesium in the system is shown in muscle cramps, irregular movements, irritability and hyperexcitability. Magnesium has been of benefit to recovering heart patients, and its use is now being investigated for epileptic cases.

The loss of magnesium, which is increased by diuretics (since magnesium is soluble in water), causes fatigue and weakness. Just as plants have magnesium at the center of their chlorophyll molecule, man has magnesium in his hemoglobin and makes use of the sun's energy much the same as the plant kingdom does for photosynthesis. Chlorophyll is essential to all of us, for it heals wounds, protects against infection, helps strengthen the acid-alkaline balance in the system, allows the skin to use vitamin D and calcium, and is also a body deodorant.

Magnesium is found in all green plants. Epsom salt (magnesium sulfate) has 10 per cent of its weight in magnesium. The need for magnesium is around half a gram per day, but it varies with the intake of calcium, phosphorus and vitamin D. A quarter of a teaspoonful of magnesium per day supplies the usual needs of a person.

Magnesium also regulates the metabolism of calcium and vitamin C; therefore it has control over all of the neuro-muscular system of the body. Several enzymatic reactions depend on the presence of magnesium to be effective. This mineral should not be forgotten when buying vitamin supplements.

POTASSIUM

Potassium is the most important element inside the cell. It counterbalances the action of sodium outside the cell in maintaining the right concentration and amount of fluids in the tissues. When this concentration is not in balance, we have a myriad of problems such as tissue swelling, vertigo (loss of balance), heartbeat irregularities and allergies. Loss of potassium causes weakness in muscle contraction, which also affects the heart muscles and the peristalsis of the intestine needed to evacuate the colon. Too much salt (sodium) in the diet leads to losses of potassium. Diuretics also deplete potassium in the system because the kidney function will not differentiate between sodium and potassium and the most soluble elements are first to be eliminated. This happens to potassium, which when lost must be replenished by potassium supplements. Lengthy losses of potassium can be fatal, as seen in prolonged cases of diarrhea.

Good food sources of potassium are fruit and vegetables and also salt substitutes which may contain more than 50 per cent potassium chloride. Potassium is restricted to prescriptions in this country, since precise needs must be evaluated by a physician. The daily requirements vary between 5 and 15 grains, depending on salt intake and general physical condition. The dosage has to be carefully adjusted, for weak doses of potassium will stimulate muscle contraction and strong doses will depress it. Too much potassium can cause colic in babies and this colic will get worse if the babies are fed baby foods which use potassium as preservative. Allergists are now looking into the use of potassium chloride to control hay fever and related symptoms.

SODIUM

Sodium maintains the proper concentration of the body fluids in the tissues outside the cells. It helps nutrition by drawing nutrients through the intestinal wall for absorption in the blood. Usually sodium is in ample supply in the body; in fact, the problem is in having too much sodium. This is often seen in cases of high blood pressure and edema (water retention in the tissues). Some cases of obesity are really water retention, and those people who go on diets will lose a lot at first because of the loss of water; they should not claim victory until they have a lasting constant weight, which can only be maintained through regular dieting and exercise. Too much sodium also depletes potassium in the tissues, which leads to fatigue, muscle cramps, irregular heartbeat and constipation. Using diuretics will eliminate all the water soluble elements such as sodium, but potassium will also be lost, causing weakness and muscle fatigue. Supplementing potassium then becomes necessary and is the usual procedure nowadays when taking diuretics. Sodium is lost in perspiration, diarrhea and vomiting and should be replaced, usually by adding salt to the drinking water; without it, heat cramps and fatigue set in.

The best source of sodium is table salt, preferably iodized. The needs are around one-half ounce, and vegetarians should watch this carefully, since their diet does not supply that amount regularly.

ZINC

The role of zinc in the system parallels the function of vitamin B-1. Zinc contributes to the formation and maturation of all body cells. It enters into the chemistry of many enzymatic reactions and specifically is essential to protein metabolism and assimilation of carbohydrates. The daily needs are consistent, for zinc is not recovered like iron in the reabsorption mechanism. The needs for zinc are around 15 mg daily.

Good food sources of zinc are liver, beans, green vegetables and other vegetables, which should be organically grown. Zinc may be absent in unorganically grown vegetables because the soil, being depleted of humus, does not have zinc in solution to be absorbed by the plant. The use of chemical fertilizers as opposed to natural organic ones causes humus to be absent in the soil, and we have one more offense against nature.

Because zinc is essential to cell formation it is needed for healing and maintenance of healthy tissues. By assuring adequate zinc intake, we increase our resistance to infections and avoid countless skin disorders of the allergy and eczema type. Zinc ointment has been a good skin healer for generations, and a lotion of zinc sulfate is currently used for acne. Undoubtedly, the local use of zinc has been proved beneficial, but the general internal action of this element is also of benefit to all other tissues in the body. It is in fact the salt of choice for some insulin preparations, and it is more widely present and in higher concentrations in the body than any other element with the exception of iron. Again, vitamin-mineral supplements should be considered when buying vitamins.

SULPHUR

Sulphur enters the formula of proteins and of their important amino acids. It acts to mature and maintain normal healthy cells, along with the bile and vitamin B-1, and carries several enzymatic reactions to their completion. The lack of sulphur is shown in brittle nails and splitting hair.

Sulphur is used topically in ointments, lotions and powders for its germicidal, fungicidal and keratolytic actions. The old Sulphur and Cream of Tartar used as blood purifier is outmoded and ineffective for that purpose. Overusage of sulphur in the soil is also a high contributor in killing the humus needed to keep minerals in solution for the plants to absorb.

Good sources of sulphur in foods are complete proteins, egg yolks, wheat germ, clams, peanuts and beef meat.

3

Foods

All foods can be classified into three categories: proteins, fats and carbohydrates. This chapter will discuss each and its effects on bodily functions.

PROTEINS

Proteins are the very substance which constitutes the major part of the cells and tissues in the body. Proteins cannot be stored to any great extent in the system so their need in nutrition is constant. Because they are essential to the growth and maintenance of healthy tissues our diet should consistently supply us with adequate amounts. Proteins are in fact responsible in delaying the aging process, for, if we don't receive enough from our diet, the body will replenish its supply from our very own tissues. This would undermine our reserves and reduce our stamina and available energy needed in times of stress, which could lead to a general debility.

The value of a protein depends on its content of amino acids. Amino acids are the active part of a protein remaining after digestion. Each amino acid has a specific role in nutrition; this role is still the object of investigation and may hold the answer to many diseases, even to certain cancers linked with cell division and tissue differentiation.

Amino acids are all essential, although they have been classified into essential and non-essential, which is misleading. The essential amino acids are those which have to be supplied by foods, since the body cannot manufacture them. The non-essential amino acids can be synthesized by the body but are just as important as the so-called essential. Combinations of different proteins form the multitude of different tissues which constitute our bodies.

Proteins are complete when they contain the following essential amino acids: leucine, isoleucine, lysine, methionine, phenylalanine, threonine, tryptophane and valine. The source of a protein may be animal or vegetable, but when you buy protein supplements check the content of amino acids. This information should be listed on the label by any reputable manufacturer; if there is no such list, you may get much less than what you pay for. Certain foods have complete proteins, such as milk, cottage cheese, yogurt, lean meat, fish, poultry, egg yolks, brewer's yeast, soybean flour and soybeans, wheat germ, American or Swiss cheese and skim milk, to name a few. Breakfast cereals are truly expensive foods which are incomplete and have almost no value in nutrition except for the milk you drink with them. I suggest you read the labels; the current trend is to add vitamins so as to divert your attention away from the low protein, high fat and carbohydrate content.

Should your diet be low in protein, the storage of amino acids in the liver will be depleted. Your more active tissues will draw their necessary amino acids from less vital body tissues, thus accelerating the aging process. You will also experience weight loss, edema (tissue swelling), low stamina, skin changes, slow healing of wounds leading to nephrosis and lowered resistance to infections, since phagocytes and leukocytes need proteins for their formation.

One very important function of protein is to maintain the blood glucose at a regular level. This action is discussed more fully in this chapter under hypoglycemia. This condition affects more people than they realize and is hard to detect. Many people have asked me for a good vitamin because they were always tired in mid-morning or mid-afternoon; my suggestion was a small thin steak for breakfast, an almost unthinkable menu. The result was astonishing; within three days these same people skipped lunch and, except for an occasional cup of tea or coffee, had found enough vigor to last them until dinnertime. Don't overrule this suggestion: it has worked for others, why not for you? The idea is to increase protein intake to five ounces per day.

Too much protein in the diet is undesirable, for amino acids are acidic and would cause a decrease in the alkali reserve of the body. This reserve is responsible for the body's stamina, a fact athletes are highly aware of. The acid-base balance of the system could be upset by too much protein in the diet; that is, the nitrogen of the proteins would be eliminated at the kidney level and the build up of glycogen would oversupply the body needs and turn into fat. This is a waste of food and an abuse of bodily functions. For these reasons, proteins must be included in the diet on a regular basis but never in excess.

FATS

Fats supply the energy needed by the human body to function. They insulate the body against temperature changes, lubricate the muscles, give support to the vital organs (lungs, kidneys), help digest other foods and also act as vehicle and storage for the oil soluble vitamins.

In the process of being digested, fats yield glycerol and fatty acids. Some fatty acids are essential to growth and the maintenance of health. This is why the two most important fatty acids, linoleic and linolenic, are called essential fatty acids. They contribute the necessary fats to the cell structure, they provide the right medium for intestinal bacterias to perform, and they also enter into the production of sex hormones. Good food sources of these essential fatty acids are mainly in vegetable oils such as corn, safflower, soya and wheat germ as well as some fish oils.

The fats which accumulate in the body and impair blood circulation are usually saturated fats of animal origin, including all dairy products, although coconut oil, coco butter and chocolate, which are of vegetable origin, also have saturated fats. These fats can be metabolized by the system from alcohol and sugar. Eventually the accumulation of these fats will show a high presence of cholesterol in the system. Lack of exercise and a constant diet of saturated fats are sure paths to high cholesterol and atherosclerosis, because the body's digestive juices cannot break down these fats. Vegetarians are less prone to this condition, for their diet is composed of unsaturated fats of vegetable origin; these fats are easily broken down into the small particles that can be used by the body cells or eliminated from the system. The National Nutrition Board advises that a diet made up of four parts of animal fat to one part of vegetable fat is an ideal ratio to avoid fat buildup in the body.

Vitamin E has been shown recently to lower cholesterol in the circulation. The optimum dose is around 300 units daily for that purpose. It is not known at what level vitamin E performs this function but its effectiveness has been measured chemically by the percentage of dienes present in the blood. Because fats are essential to life and growth, it is up to us to select vegetable unsaturated fats and oils in preference to fats of animal origin. Apart from increasing vegetable fat intake in the diet, the use of vitamin E will break down the already accumulated saturated fats into smaller particles that can either be used by the cells or eliminated. The benefits are many. Lower cholesterol and a better blood circulation will never be seen, but some effects are obvious: Eczemas often respond to vitamin E, frequent burning during urination is relieved, repeated colds and sore throats diminish, seborrhea (dandruff) is corrected, ulcers and colitis are often healed and cured.

The Food and Drug Administration, in December 1971, began a major initiative to improve the nutritional labeling of food products. Of most interest is a proposed change in fat labeling. The F.D.A. has proposed regulations requiring product labels to give the name, source and amount of fat content and, on some foods, the amount and kind of fatty acids present. Under this proposal such uninformative labeling as "shortening" or "vegetable oil" would cease. It is the intention of the F.D.A. to make it possible for the buyer to determine the nutritional value of the food he is buying by reading the label.

CARBOHYDRATES

The chemistry of carbohydrates is essentially that of sugar, candy, cake, starches, bread, jam, pastries and potatoes, to name a few. In the digestive process they are all broken down into their simplest element: sugar. Carbohydrates provide instant energy and if the diet provides us with more energy than we can use, it is stored mainly in the liver as glycogen, available for later demands of energy. Lack of this capacity to release glycogen when needed causes hypoglycemia, which will be treated later in this chapter. Should the storage of glycogen reach its full capacity, any more carbohydrates will become fat and obesity will result.

Lack of exercise and oversupply of carbohydrates or alcohol (sugar) are the main causes of high cholesterol and weight gain. This condition taxes the heart in its work of supplying blood where needed. Every eight pounds of excess body weight is like carrying a gallon of water day and night.

Carbohydrates also impair the absorption of iron, which might result in anemia. Calcium absorption is also impaired by overpresence of carbohydrates, since calcium requires a lot of the stomach acid monopolized by carbohydrates during digestion. This is why sweets affect the teeth (by impairing calcium absorption). The needs for the B complex vitamins are also increased when carbohydrates are high in the diet, for their metabolism cannot be effected without these vitamins; this is evident in the treatment of alcoholism where the B complex vitamins are used to detoxicate a person with a hangover. The appetite is also impaired, for carbohydrates use up most of the gastric juices and the insulin available, thus suppressing hunger for other more nutritive foods.

Carbohydrates do appeal to the taste buds but are a sure way to obesity and malnutrition. Here is a list of the big offenders: cookies, breakfast cereals, custards, pies, sweet sauces, cocoa, soft drinks, gum, dried fruits, fruit cocktails, syrup, coconut, ice cream and sherbets. Where can you cut your diet without upsetting the balance necessary for good nutrition? The answer should not be hard; start with carbohydrates.

CHOLESTEROL

Cholesterol is a necessary constituent of the cells and also enters into the synthesis of certain hormones. But cholesterol in excessive concentration in the blood has been found to clog up the capillaries (small blood vessels) as well as accumulate along the arterial walls, causing coronary occlusions and a stroke if the plaques should become loose in the circulation. These strokes can well cause paralysis and even death, for the brain can be affected to a greater or lesser degree.

The major cause of high concentrations of cholesterol in the blood is a diet rich in animal meats and dairy products. But other products such as the poisons in your

food known as insecticides, conditioners, dyes, preservatives, buffers, thickeners, extenders, bleaches, sweeten-
ers (remember the cyclamates) and others—all cause a
little bit more oxidation in your system, sometimes to the
point of no return. A high level of cholesterol indicates a
high risk of heart disease, and since the oxidation products of cholesterol are carcinogenic (cancer causing), it
goes without saying that these cholesterol-containing
foods should be eaten in moderation.

Besides restricting foods of animal origin (including
dairy products), one should increase the intake of foods
of vegetable origin in the diet. The problem with cholesterol is its overabundance in normal diets. The national
average intake is around 600 mg daily, and the needs
normally are about 300 mg. Since one egg yolk supplies
230 to 275 mg of cholesterol, it is easy to see how we can
have an oversupply. The chemistry of animal fats and
dairy products is such that they form saturated fats and
cholesterol in the system. A few products of vegetable
origin, such as coconut oil and chocolate products, also
form saturated fats and should be limited in the diet. The
above are general rules but here are some specifics:

Do not fry eggs; boil them and limit them to three per
week.
Eat your breakfast cereals (if you are addicted) with
low fat milk.
Drink your coffee black or use skim milk. Use little or
no sugar.
Bacon has no value in nutrition; ham is a good substitute.

Sausage and bologna should be ruled out.

Fish is as nutritive as meat and offers variety.

Don't fry meats. Use the barbecue or the broiler. That fat must be taken out.

Use oil-vinegar salad dressings instead of complicated creamy sauces and dressings. This will increase vegetable oil in your diet.

Eat more fresh vegetables and fruits.

Finally, if you really want to feel the difference, you can take 300 units of vitamin E in your diet each day. This will reduce the cholesterol in your system to the finer particle size which can be utilized by the cells or eliminated. Allow two weeks for a marked improvement but results should be felt within three or four days.

COMMON SENSE IN YOUR DIET

Nutritionists and medical experts are still divided sharply over conflicting facts about foods and diets. The greatest damage is often done at the dinner table; but what changes in eating habits will give the most benefit? Will avoiding one food stave off a heart attack or prevent atherosclerosis? Is the sacrifice worth it? The problem is prominent because over half a million Americans die of coronaries each year and countless others limit their activities for fear of precipitating a heart attack. All this because they choose the wrong foods. The American Medical Association and the Food and Drug Administration cannot guarantee that a change in the diet will be of benefit, although strong indications point to it.

Cholesterol is the big offender and nutritionists have

been alerted to the problem for about twenty years. More data is needed to confirm already strong opinions. Atherosclerosis attacks young people increasingly, because invariably there is a high amount of cholesterol in their blood. This hypercholesterolemia, as it is called, causes roughening of the walls of the arteries and leads to the narrowing of these vessels; hence there is a decrease of blood supply vital to the heart, lungs and the brain. Should the plaques of cholesterol that have clung to the walls of the arteries become loosened and travel in the circulatory system, they may cause a heart stroke or a brain hemorrhage.

How can you play it safe without sacrificing all the pleasures of tasty foods? Americans are big meat eaters; by contrast, the Japanese are mainly fish eaters. When studies were made on Japanese immigrants who had increased the amount of meat in their diet, they were found to have a much higher cholesterol level than before.

The change in diet necessary to avoid this situation is simple and effective. Typically, an increase in vegetable oil up to five tablespoonfuls daily blended with other foods or juices or used in salad dressings would be ideal. Unsaturated vegetable oils such as corn oil, safflower or soybean oils are suitable. The increase in unsaturated fats coupled with a decrease in animal fats and dairy products will show a marked reduction in cholesterol. If you happen to be on a reducing program these unsaturated fats will also reduce the saturated fats accumulated in your body. Chemically, it works, and the results will be steady and lasting.

The quantity of meat should be limited to four ounces

of lean beef, pork or lamb every other day. Alternate these main dishes with sea foods and poultry meat. Increase your consumption of vegetables, but avoid starch-containing potatoes. Have more salads with oil-vinegar dressings. Drink skim milk and avoid all dairy products, except cottage cheese, because of their high content of cholesterol. Fruits and fruit juices are recommended. Avoid coconut, chocolate, ice cream and sherbet. Cake mixes, egg yolks, bacon fat, chicken skin are not recommended.

One last word. The next time you go food shopping look around and compare how obese people have their shopping carts loaded with fattening foods, while thin people do the very opposite. There has to be a reason; maybe you know why.

CALORIES

Calorie has become a superword in the language of dieters; in fact, at one time, before vitamins became popular, your neighborhood drugstore would feature calorie tablets promising energy, zest, vigor, etc., all in the name of good health. It is a wise thing to count calories and the physically active worker will undoubtedly need and burn more calories than an office worker. Therefore, food requirements vary with physical activity, age, sex and size. If your food supplies more calories than you can burn, there is no doubt that you will gain weight. Yet, calories are not the whole answer to weight problems. A balanced diet and regular exercise still remain the most effective ways to control weight.

Of course, the food industry saw a dollar to be made in that field. Liquid diets in cans guarantee good health and weight loss without effort. To this day I know of no one who could carry on with those diets and achieve their purpose. Sluggishness becomes predominant, constipation sets in and irritability develops. Eventually, the dieter gives up altogether.

The answer to weight problems resides in a change in eating habits while maintaining balanced nutrition. At first, reducing the quantity of food your stomach is used to receive could challenge your will power; after three or four days your stomach won't "shrink" but your digestive juices will be secreted in smaller amounts and your hunger will be satisfied with less food. Above all, don't fill up with soups or other liquids; this merely dilutes your gastric juices and gives no lasting satisfaction. Instead, prepare salads or other blends, preferably of vegetable origin, so as to supply the bulk needed to maintain your peristalsis and avoid constipation. Your main dish especially should supply proteins to make use of your appetite and avoid the burning of your own tissues as the source of proteins. Chew each mouthful thoroughly, as this allows your salivary enzymes to mix well and digest your foods more completely. Do not fry your foods, for this adds extra calories and saturated fats which you are trying to avoid. Don't use creamy and complicated sauces in salad dressings; restrict your needs to oil-vinegar. Do use tomatoes, celery, cucumber, cabbage and other vegetables, for they are full of minerals and vitamins and contribute to the taste and variety of the menu. Try using skim milk in your coffee and skip the sugar (maybe you've forgotten the true taste of coffee). You can use saccharin if you must, but not in excessive amounts, for it is damaging to the urinary system, especially the bladder. Snacks should be made of fruits and cottage cheese, not candies or cookies. A light lunch also made up of cottage cheese or other protein and fresh fruit will supply nutrition and satisfy your appetite until dinnertime. Gelatin desserts are poor suppliers of proteins but are low in calories.

HYPOGLYCEMIA

This condition, which has the opposite effects and symptoms of diabetes, means that there is too little sugar in the blood. Even a complete physical exam may fail to show the presence of this condition. This is why you may be hypoglycemic and not be aware of it, although it may affect you mentally as well as physically. Once diagnosed, it can be relieved in most cases, but you will have to live with it, since there is no sure cure. Some remissions do occur, just as quickly as the sickness itself sets in, without any warning.

The immediate cause of hypoglycemia seems to be in a faulty carbohydrate metabolism; the pancreas and the liver don't release a steady flow of glucose (glycogen) into the blood. This result is shown in sudden bursts of energy, usually after eating, followed by periods of sluggishness. The symptoms are many: in children, hypoglycemia causes a lack of concentration paired with physical hyperactivity and gradual development of sleeplessness. Adults also have bursts of energy followed by lassitude, and they are short tempered. They wake up just as tired as when they went to bed; everything is an effort; rashes may develop and trembling may set in. Daydreaming, lack of interest and concentration and unfounded fears may be present. You may have had sessions of that sort not knowing why "you were not yourself that day" or why you treated that person or that event in such a silly way. To this day you can't explain why you were not yourself. All the symptoms may have been present for some time or may have appeared quite suddenly. If you can't put your finger on the cause, you may well have had hypoglycemia all along. As a matter of fact, psychiatrists have been aware of the problem for some time now; some emotionally disturbed patients have been found to have hypoglycemia. Psychiatrists insist on a glucose tolerance test on suspected patients.

We are now learning more and more that our chemistry makes us what we are, mentally as well as physically. Consider the pioneering work of Linus Pauling when he investigated schizophrenics who retain vitamin C in their system while most people do not. He found a definite relationship established between mental and physical factors.

The release of glucose in the blood is controlled by the adrenal glands, and the glucose is stored in the liver and to a lesser extent in the tissues themselves. When not enough glucose is available, we experience hunger. Under normal conditions, the level of glucose in the blood is maintained at 100 mg per 100 cc of blood. This balance is maintained by the insulin and regulated by the adrenals. Such is not the case for hypoglycemics, where the storage of glycogen is small and the glucose from the food gets used up as soon as it is released in digestion. This situation creates frequent hunger usually satisfied by sweets and stimulants such as coffee. Again the cycle is repeated, and we have a vicious series of ups and downs after each meal and every snack throughout the day. A dreadful weight gain ensues, although the calories consumed may be less than 1500 per day. From then on, the patient does not know where to turn, and if he should see a physician who suspects hypoglycemia, he should be thankful and go through with the test. The expense and trouble are worth it, because if he shows negative, he will know that much more and his doctor can look for something else that might be wrong.

In a glucose tolerance test, a sample of your blood is collected before the test and the glucose content is measured. You are given a glucose cocktail containing a measured amount of glucose, and samples of your blood are then collected hourly for four or five hours for analysis. The results will indicate whether you metabolise your glucose in a steady fashion, or whether you show irregular patterns of glucose in your blood.

Every living cell in the body needs glucose to function. The need is constant, so glucose must be at a normal level constantly; otherwise the mental and physical balance of the whole system is threatened and can become unstable.

Many children of school age were diagnosed as hyperkinetic (overactive), sometimes by a teacher who, for the sake of "peace in the classroom," would request the parents to use tranquilizers or the popular Ritalin. The parent often complied without question, not realizing that the child's problem was hypoglycemia. Frankly, some of the teachers should be on Valium or Premarin themselves, for their "solution" could ruin a child's personality forever.

How do we deal with hypoglycemia? The latest practice is to increase protein intake at mealtime, for protein gives a sustained release of glycogen, while the blood sugar can be supported between meals with protein-carbohydrate foods. Frequent feedings can be avoided if proteins form the major part of the food. A high protein breakfast would include eggs (watch out for cholesterol) and ham or even steak; tea instead of coffee, for coffee stimulates the adrenals which release glucose; one slice of toast (well buttered); and orange or grapefruit or their juices. In midmorning, a good food would be cottage cheese, which is a complete protein, with a fresh fruit. For lunch, meat or fish with a lightly cooked vegetable, little or no bread, and no sugar with tea (not coffee). The afternoon snack could include milk and cottage cheese or a fresh fruit or fruit salad without syrup or cheese and nuts. Dinner can alternate between fish, meat or poultry with a green vegetable, little or no bread, and milk or tea without sugar.

From the above, you can see that sugar is not allowed, for sugar undermines the supplies of the B vitamins and requires more energy to burn than it produces, so sugar represents empty calories. Sugar is found in canned fruit cocktails, fruit juices, soft drinks, sweet fruits, sherbet and others. Allowed fruits include lemons, oranges, melons, avocados, apricots, pineapple, grapefruits and peaches. Starchy vegetables such as potatoes and peas are to be avoided, but vegetables of the green type, such as asparagus, broccoli, celery, cauliflower, spinach, squash, cabbage, tomatoes and turnip, are encouraged. Coffee and cola drinks have caffeine, which acclerates the burning of glycogen and depletes the supply too quickly. Also not allowed are pastries, sweets, spaghetti, macaroni and the sweet fruits such as pears, grapes, dates, figs, apples and bananas.

There is one vitamin which has been shown valuable for hypoglycemics. I am speaking of pantothenic acid, which increases the capacity of the liver to store glycogen. This vitamin belongs to the B complex group and is truly an anti-stress vitamin. It acts mainly in slowing down the breakdown of proteins. A daily dose of 100 mg taken two or three times is average. Athletes have made good use of this vitamin to increase their stamina. Other vitamins of the B complex should also be supplied, because of their involvement in glucose metabolism.

FOOD SHOPPING

For most of us, good nutrition starts at the food market. By now you should be familiar with proteins, carbohydrates, fats, polyunsaturates, starches, amino acids and other classes of foods and their contents. You are aware of vitamins and minerals and you are therefore in a position to shop more intelligently, because pretty labels and colorful wrappings are now meaningless; you are a label reader, and if the wrapper on foods does not clearly state the contents, you won't buy it. You might even go as far as to write the manufacturer to question the content of his product. Even the largest food manufacturers will skip mentioning the large amount of fats and carbohydrates, but when the protein content is high, you can be sure that the same manufacturer will take pride and mention it on the label. The F.D.A. has done some good work in this area lately; the labeling of fats and vegetable oils will now show the percentage, origin and actual content of saturated or hydrogenated fats and oils. This is a step in the right direction.

With the advent of pre-cooked foods you may have become a constant user of can openers, thus underestimating your own capacity as a chef. You are giving in to a bad habit, because you could eat better for less money.

Meats are a major item in the food budget. Fat means cholesterol, so you will probably avoid meat cuts with thick layers of fat which outweigh the meat by two to one, and since it is saturated, you want it out before you eat it. You will also avoid meat interlarded with fat; you will select leaner cuts. You will buy ground round instead of ground beef; you will buy sirloin roast instead of a fat rib roast. Don't disregard fish and poultry, for these meats offer nearly pure proteins besides adding variety to the menu. Fresh fruits and vegetables supply vitamins, minerals and other nutritive factors; don't overlook them in preference to less tasty and less nutritious canned equivalents.

Frozen dinners are very expensive; if you compare the net weight with similar fresh unfrozen foods, the price may be four times as much, and they contain additives, colorings, preservatives, thickeners, bleaches, etc., which you should be leary of. Cake mixes may eventually have their contents listed on their labels. Margarines are to be preferred over butter, and the unsaturated margarines

are of better value. Lard and shortening are saturated
fats, and nothing less.

Try using low-fat or non-fat milk whenever possible
in coffee, cereals and cooking in general; every little bit
of fat intake adds up. The regular use of oil-vinegar as
salad dressing over complicated sauces will contribute to
the higher intake of unsaturated vegetable oils and avoid
one more cholesterol-containing ingredient.

Now that you have invested sound thinking in selecting
healthier foods at the supermarket, you may not feel too
badly when you pay the cashier, for it's not just a money
matter; some wisdom went into it.

FOODS AND NATURE

The coming of colorful packagings and labels has steered
us away from fresh natural foods. Fruits and vegetables
are now canned, frozen, pre-cooked, ready-to-eat, preserved, dyed and, worst of all, grown on soils deprived of
minerals and loaded with insecticides and other chemicals. These foods used to be grown organically (like in
the olden days) and not forced to ripen artificially. To
improve your health or just to maintain your health, you
must make some changes in your eating habits. Feeding
habits should vary with age, profession, weight and health
condition.

Avoid canned foods, for they are heated, preserved, colored, thickened, bleached, flavored, dyed, buffered, sweet-
ened and conditioned and will oxidize your system, accelerating cell destruction and contributing to premature
aging. Literally, canned foods will disrupt the delicate
balance of your body chemistry. Avoid animal meats and

dairy products because of their cholesterol content, and increase your consumption of fruits and vegetables. Fish and poultry will give you as much protein as animal meat without the cholesterol content, and your kidney function won't be overburdened as it is by meat; your liver will also benefit from this treatment. Never fry meats, instead, broil or barbecue them in order to eliminate the saturated fats they contain. Avoid also heavy foods such as fried potatoes, creamy sauces and salad dressings. Avoid cakes, cookies and pastries, for they are hard to digest and contain no proteins. Buy 100 per cent whole wheat bread, because white bread has 70 different chemicals added to it before it reaches you. Milk should be of the low-fat, non-fat or skimmed variety. Yogurt should be eaten daily, for it favors intestinal fermentation and the elaboration of countless vitamins and enzymes; it also helps metabolism and absorption of vitamin C.

Natural spices can be used in moderation but chemical aromatics should be avoided. The constant use of meat tenderizers is not advisable, for if they act on meat, they will also act on the tissues in the digestive system. They also digest some of the vitamin B complex group; prolonged use of digestive enzymes is therefore not recommended.

Another major cause of chemistry imbalance in the body is alcohol, especially the straight drinks, which literally dissolve the protective fats and oils of the digestive system; this is a sure way to ulcers and flatulence. Beer and wine are much more tolerable. Alcohol imposes a heavy demand for vitamin B to be metabolized, which undermines the body supplies, decreases stamina and dulls the brain. The effects on the kidney and liver functions and on the reproductive organs are not to be understated. The coagulating action of alcohol on the blood tends to impair circulation; it hardens the arteries and, because it turns to sugar, it elevates the cholesterol level.

Avoid smoking, for if you smoke you cannot be healthy. I am not referring only to cancer but to the multitude of respiratory and digestive disturbances which slowly undermine your health. The problem with smokers is that they take their health for granted, and even when they have emphysema, bronchitis, asthma and palpitations, they come to the drugstore with a cigarette in their mouth. Women did not become habit smokers until some 20 years after men did, and now all the ill effects of smoking are showing up in women. If you smoke you owe yourself a favor. But maybe you owe your young son or daughter a favor, for after all *you* brought them into this world. Don't smoke, and live longer.

EATING HABITS

Variety at mealtime may help food enjoyment, but digesting an assortment of foods may sometimes place a burden on the system, since different foods are digested at different places along the digestive tract. Granted you may digest each food separately, but the combination in one meal of several dishes may present a problem, for some foods just don't go together. This is a very individual thing and those who have "strong stomachs" can enjoy these strange combinations, at least for some time, but trouble may eventually show up. Chewing one food usually triggers the release of digestive sugars in the stomach and intestine, for that food will eventually reach that level of digestion and need this specific sugar for its metabolism. Here are food combinations to avoid:

Don't eat sweet fruit and bitter fruit together (they require different sugars and different mediums to be digested).

Don't combine sweet fruits and vegetables (your digestive sugars will be diluted beyond their digesting capacity).

Don't eat bitter fruits with proteins or starches (they require different mediums and different digestive enzymes which are incompatible).

Don't combine watermelon, honeydew or cantalope with any other food (they inhibit the action of your digestive juices).

Don't use sugar on fresh fruit (sugar contains empty calories which will prevent the absorption of the fruit itself).

Don't eat sweets with starchy foods (both require enormous amounts of pepsin and diastase in an acid medium to digest properly).

Don't combine proteins with starchy foods.

Don't eat fat foods with protein foods.

Don't combine two kinds of starchy foods in one meal.

Proteins go well with green vegetables, but not with potatoes or other starches. Starchy foods (rice, potatoes) go well with green vegetables (raw or lightly cooked). Chewing takes care of half of your digestion for it physically breaks the food and mixes it with the salivary enzymes and sugars needed for assimilation. Most ulcers start from faulty chewing. Never eat when upset, for you can't absorb nutrition under tension. Try to eat your bigger meals early in the day when you need the energy and can burn the calories; at night your calories may not be burned and will turn to fat, and might disturb your sleep.

THE AGING PROCESS

Because aging is highly controlled by the oxidation (burning) of the cells, please refer to the section on vitamin E, which applies to this topic of aging.

There are two or three natural products which I want to mention here, for they are undervalued and truly inexpensive and natural. I am referring to honey, natural vinegar and lemon, which have been used routinely in Vermont; this state claims to have the highest average of longevity in the U.S.

Honey

Honey has the vitamins A, B-1, B-2, C, K and E and niacin; it also has Copper, Magnesium, Iron, Calcium, Iodine, Manganese, Potassium, Tin, Boron and other minerals. It is antiseptic, for it contains formic acid; it is a natural sugar, for 95 per cent of it is glucose and so provides instant energy. Honey is predigested by the bee; therefore it is well tolerated by diabetics in moderate amounts. Honey helps healing and increases resistance to infections. Taken before meals with cold water it increases the quantity of digestive sugars and after meals in hot water it decreases acidity. It relieves constipation in babies and children. During the cold months, honey is an excellent substitute for jam on toast in the morning. It helps prevent colds by keeping the digestive tract aseptic. Honey is truly one of the most perfect foods.

Vinegar

Natural vinegar, which is brown and fermented naturally from apples and wine, contains an abundance of vitamins and minerals. It acts in restoring the acid-base balance of the system and in this way increases stamina and mental alertness. Vinegar improves memory, promotes healing, reduces arthritis, increases capillary circulation and regulates body heat. Vinegar improves calcium absorption from the food while it rids the calcium deposits which impair the bone movements in the joints.

The combination of one tablespoonful of natural vinegar and honey, taken in hot water and sipped slowly to mix it thoroughly with the saliva, is the old secret formula from Vermont. This can be repeated morning and night. Lemon juice freshly extracted from the lemon can be substituted for the vinegar, and has shown good results in many a case of arthritis and rheumatism. There it is if you want to use it; some old folks from Vermont swear by it.

4

Poisons and Poisonous Plants

Grateful acknowledgment is made to the California State Board of Pharmacy and to its Poisons and Antidote Committee for the permission granted to reproduce in part the updated Official California Antidotes and First Aid Treatments. The use of certain trade names is restricted to the misuse of such products and does not refer to their normal toxicity.

GENERAL MEASURES

The following sixteen treatments are for immediate use after an accident. Seeking help from the fire department while awaiting a physician is good thinking. Do not undervalue the fire department, for they have wireless communications besides their own equipment and qualifications.

TREATMENT NO. 1: If conscious, give tap water. Then induce vomiting by touching the back of the throat or giving one teaspoonful of salt in a glass of warm water. Repeat until vomit fluid is clear. If not breathing: Use artificial respiration. Keep patient warm and quiet.

TREATMENT NO. 2: INTERNAL: Give tap water, milk of magnesia or eggs beaten in water. EXTERNAL: Wash with running water, then with water containing baking soda.

TREATMENT NO. 3: If conscious, give tap water and induce vomiting. Repeat until vomit fluid is clear. Keep patient warm and quiet. If not breathing, use artificial respiration and then give strong tea or coffee.

TREATMENT NO. 4: If conscious, give tap water and induce vomiting until vomit fluid is clear. Give two teaspoonfuls of baking soda in water. Protect the eyes from light. Use artificial respiration if needed. Keep patient warm and quiet. Give strong tea or coffee.

TREATMENT NO. 5: IN THE EYES: Wash with a stream of water, holding the lids open. Then wash with a solution of boric acid. ON THE SKIN: Flood with plenty of water, then wash with vinegar. INTERNAL: Give water with large amounts of diluted vinegar, lemon or orange juice. Then give eggs beaten in water, or give milk. Keep warm and quiet. Use artificial respiration if needed.

TREATMENT NO. 6: If conscious, give tap water and induce vomiting until vomit fluid is clear. Keep patient calm.

TREATMENT NO. 7: If conscious, give tap water and induce vomiting until vomit fluid is clear. Give milk or egg whites beaten in water. Keep warm and quiet.

TREATMENT NO. 8: If conscious, give tap water and induce vomiting until vomit fluid is clear. Protect eyes from light. Apply ice packs and cooling baths. Keep calm and quiet.

TREATMENT NO. 9: Move victim to fresh air and use artificial respiration if needed. If the poison has been swallowed and the patient is conscious, give tap water and induce vomiting until vomit fluid is clear.

TREATMENT NO. 10: If conscious, give tap water and induce vomiting until vomit fluid is clear. Give starch paste, mashed potatoes, milk or eggs beaten in water. Keep patient warm and quiet.

TREATMENT NO. 11: Use artificial respiration if needed. If conscious, give tap water and induce vomiting until vomit fluid is clear. Give four ounces of mineral oil, if available. Give large amounts of warm water.

TREATMENT NO. 12: Give tap water and induce vomiting until vomit fluid is clear. Then give a tablespoonful of salt dissolved in a quart of water. Give plenty of water and then give strong tea or coffee.

TREATMENT NO. 13: If conscious, give tap water and induce vomiting until vomit fluid is clear. Give one tablespoonful of baking soda dissolved in a quart of water. Keep patient warm and quiet.

TREATMENT NO. 14: Move patient to fresh air and use artificial respiration if needed.

TREATMENT NO. 15: INTERNAL: Give tap water, then milk, milk of magnesia or eggs beaten in water. EXTERNAL: Wash with tap water, flood with alcohol, then wash with soap and water.

TREATMENT NO. 16: Move victim to fresh air and use
   artificial respiration if needed. If poison was swallowed,
   do not induce vomiting.

INDEX TO FIRST AID TREATMENTS (THE NUMBERS REFER TO THE ABOVE TREATMENTS)

Borax	6	Cleaning fluid	16, 9
Boric acid	6	Clove oil	11
Bromates	3	Cocaine	1
Bromides	3	Codeine	3
Bromine	2	Collyrium (eye wash)	6
Bromo Seltzer	1, 3	Contac	8
Burrows Solution	7	Copper compounds	7
Butane	16	Coumadin	6
Butisol	3	Crayons	1
Caffeine	1	Creosote	15
Campho phenique	6, 15	Cresol	15
Camphor	6	Cuticle remover	5
Camphorated oil	6	Cyanides	3
Cannabis	6	DDT	9
Canned heat	4	Dent's ear drops	3
Carbolic acid	15	Dexedrine	6
Carbon monoxide	14	Dichloramine-T	3
Carbon disulfide	9	Dichloricide	9
Carbon tetrachloride	9	Dichloro phenol	9
Cascara or cascara sagrada	1	Dicoumarol	6
Castor beans	7	Dinitro-orthocresol	8
Caustic pencils	12	Dinitrophenol	8
Caustic soda	5	DNTP	1
Cepacol	5	DPP	1
Chloral hydrate	3	Drano	5
Chlorates	3	Dry cleaning fluid	16, 9
Chlordane (same as DDT)	9	Dynamite	1
Chloride of Lime	5	Empirin	1
Chlorine	14	Ergot	6
Chloroform	9	Ether	9
Chlorox	5	Ethyl acetate	16
Chromates	7	Ethyl chloride	9
Chromic Acid	2	Ethyl nitrite	1
Cinnamon Oil	11	Eucalyptus oil	11
Citric acid	7	Eugenol	11
Cleaner's Benzine	16, 9	Eyelash dye	1

Quick lime	5	Sulfuric acid	2
Quinine	6	Tannic acid	15
Rat nip	11	Tansy oil	11
Roach pastes	11	Tartaric acid	2
Roach powders	7	Tartar emetic	7
Rough on rats	7	Ten-eighty	6
Saccharin	1	Thallium compounds	3
Salicylamide	1	Thinners (paint)	16
Salicylates	1	Thymol	15
Sani flush	5	Tin compounds	7
Savin oil	11	Tincture iodine	10
Selsun	1	Tintex (dyes)	1
Sheep dip	15	Tobacco	3
Shellac	4	Toluene	16
Shoe polish	1, 16	Toothpastes (fluorinated)	7
Silver compounds	12	Toxakil	9
Silver cleaners	3	Toxaphene	9
Silver nitrate	12	Two-Four-D (2-4-D)	9
Slaked lime	5	Tylenol	1
Sloans Liniment	1, 6	Valium	1
Snail baits	6, 7	Varnish	16
Soda ash	5	Vicks Rub	6
Sodium borate	6	Vince	6
Sodium cyanide	3	Water colors	1
Sodium fluoroacetate	6	Wax (floor or furniture)	16
Sodium hydroxide	5	Wintergreen oil	1
Sodium perborate	6	Wood alcohol	4
Sodium salicylate	1	Xylene	16
Solvents (volatile)	16	Xylol	16
Spanish fly	7	Xylenol	15
Spirits of Camphor	6	Zephiran	5
Spot remover	9, 16	Zinc Acetate	7
Strychnine	6	Zinch Chloride	2, 7
Sugar of lead	7	Zinc compounds	7
Sulfa drugs	13	Zinc oxide	non toxic
Sulfur chloride	2	Zirconium oxide	non toxic
Sulfur dioxide	14	Zonite	5

POISONOUS PLANTS

Numerous plants are toxic and the leaves, berries, flowers, seeds and stalks can cause pain, illness and even death. Over 10,000 cases of plant poisoning, mostly involving children, are reported each year in the U.S. Sixty per cent of those parents involved have no awareness that these plants are dangerous. If you suspect that your child has eaten some part of a toxic plant, try to save the plant for identification. Should swelling develop in or around the mouth, the tongue may swell to the point of blocking respiration; use a tongue depressor to keep the air passage clear until you get to the emergency department of the hospital. The sample of the plant can be life-saving, for the doctor will know what measures to take. Until you can reach the hospital, if nausea develops, try to save the vomit, for this also may be of value in helping to identify what the poison is.

Plants That Have Toxic Properties

Decorative Plants

AZALEAS: All parts are poisonous. Cause nausea, depress respiration, leading to coma and death.

BLEEDING HEARTS: The leaves and roots if eaten in large amounts may cause death.

CASTOR BEANS: The seeds can kill (one or two can kill an adult).

DAFFODILS: The bulbs cause nausea or vomiting and are deadly.

DAPHNE: The berries are fatal.

ELEPHANT EAR: All parts can irritate the mouth and the tongue, and swelling may block air passage in the throat.

FOXGLOVE: The leaves contain digitalis, which acts on the heart. May cause death.

GOLDEN CHAIN: The seeds (inside capsule) may cause convulsions and even death.

HYACINTH: The bulbs cause nausea, vomiting, and are deadly.

HYDRANGEAS: May be fatal from the hydrocyanic acid they contain.

IRIS: The stems can upset the digestive system.

JESSAMINE: The berries upset the stomach and may be fatal.

LARKSPUR: The seeds may be fatal.

LAURELS: All parts are poisonous. They cause nausea, depress respiration, causing coma and death.

LILY OF THE VALLEY: The leaves and flowers cause irregular heartbeat, stomach upset and mental confusion.

MISTLETOE: The berries are fatal.

OLEANDER: The leaves and branches upset the digestive tract. May cause death.

POINSETTIA: One leaf can be fatal.

RED SAGE: The green (not red) berries are fatal.

RHODODENDRONS: All parts are poisonous. They cause nausea, depress breathing, leading to coma and death.

STAR OF BETHLEHEM: The bulbs cause nausea and vomiting. Can be deadly.

WISTERIA: The seeds and pods can cause digestive disturbances.

YEW: The berries and the leaves can kill without any warning symptoms.

Vegetable and Fruit Plants

APPLE: The seeds in large amounts can cause prostration from the hydrocyanic acid they contain.

APRICOTS: The seeds may be fatal and the leaves contain hydrocyanic acid.

CHERRY: The leaves and twigs are fatal. The cyanide causes prostration within minutes.

ELDERBERRY: The leaves and shoots (used as pea shooters) can cause nausea and upset the stomach.

POTATO: The sprouts can upset the digestive tract.

RHUBARB: The leaf is fatal; eaten raw or cooked, it can cause convulsions and coma.

Shrubs and Trees

BUTTERCUPS: All parts cause deep irritation of the digestive tract.

POISON HEMLOCK: All parts are fatal. Resembles a large wild carrot.

WATER HEMLOCK: All parts cause convulsions. They are fatal.

JIMSON WEED: All parts are toxic. Causes thirst, affects vision, causes imbalance. It is responsible for a high percentage of poisonings and may be deadly.

BLACK LOCUST: The leaves and bark cause nausea and weakness.

MAYAPPLE: The roots, leaves and apple can cause diarrhea.

NIGHTSHADE: All parts cause stomach and nervous upset. Usually is fatal.

OAK: The leaves and acorns if chewed will eventually affect the kidneys.